FoodFrame

Diet is a Four-Letter Word

Risa Groux, CN

Copyright © 2021 Risa Groux, CN.

All rights reserved. No part of this book may be used or reproduced by any means, graphic, electronic, or mechanical, including photocopying, recording, taping or by any information storage retrieval system without the written permission of the author except in the case of brief quotations embodied in critical articles and reviews.

This book is a work of non-fiction. Unless otherwise noted, the author and the publisher make no explicit guarantees as to the accuracy of the information contained in this book and in some cases, names of people and places have been altered to protect their privacy.

Archway Publishing books may be ordered through booksellers or by contacting:

Archway Publishing
1663 Liberty Drive
Bloomington, IN 47403
www.archwaypublishing.com
844-669-3957

Because of the dynamic nature of the Internet, any web addresses or links contained in this book may have changed since publication and may no longer be valid. The views expressed in this work are solely those of the author and do not necessarily reflect the views of the publisher, and the publisher hereby disclaims any responsibility for them.

Any people depicted in stock imagery provided by Getty Images are models, and such images are being used for illustrative purposes only.
Certain stock imagery © Getty Images.

Interior Image Credit: Risa and Sarah Groux

ISBN: 978-1-6657-0638-4 (sc)
ISBN: 978-1-6657-0639-1 (hc)
ISBN: 978-1-6657-0640-7 (e)

Library of Congress Control Number: 2021908352

Print information available on the last page.

Archway Publishing rev. date: 10/07/2021

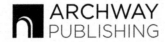

"Everyone wants to eat healthy, but people are confused when they hear about all the different diet types and ways of eating. Risa Groux, a respected holistic nutritionist, does an exceptional job defining the Low Lectin FoodFrame along with highlighting its significant benefits for improved health."

--Steven R. Gundry, MD, New York Times Bestselling Author of **The Plant Paradox**

"Risa has successfully removed the confusion from popular eating plans and defines what each person needs from each diet type in *Food Frame*. She not only explains why each person has different food needs, but she also offers delicious recipes with mouthwatering photos, that are simple and easy-to-make for whatever diet type you choose. Risa's book makes it easy to decide what to have for dinner!"

-- Josh Axe, DC, DNM, CNS, Bestselling Author of **Eat Dirt**

"Risa covers all the bases and provides delicious recipes to keep the body satisfied and free of toxins. She knows her stuff!"

-- Suzanne Somers, actress, bestselling author, singer, businesswoman, and health spokesperson

"In a quandary as to what diet you should follow? Confused with all the choices...Paleo? Keto? Vegan? Risa's got you covered, deliciously! Her personal journey with autoimmune disease led her on a path to discovering her personalized FoodFrames and now she helps you do the same in *Food Frame*. Whatever your health concerns, and your goals, you'll find the right plan for you."

-- JJ Virgin, CNS, CHFS, Celebrity Nutrition & Fitness Expert, four-time New York Times bestselling author, including **The Virgin Diet** *and* **The Sugar Impact Diet**

DEDICATION

To all my clients, past, present, and future, for your courage to gain knowledge and make the effort required to improve your health naturally. I give you all a sparkly star!

To my amazing children Sarah and Chase. You are the best part of my journey! May you always dance in the rain, sing out loud, create and earn what you want, and eat your vegetables!

Please share the gift of good health with your loved ones and make this world a healthier planet!

TABLE OF CONTENTS

INTRODUCTION - HOW HASHIMOTO'S CHANGED MY LIFE ix

PART I   IMPROVE THE WAY YOU EAT 1

Chapter 1   GROUND-FLOOR ESSENTIALS FOR HEALTH WITH EVERY EATING LIFESTYLE 3

Chapter 2   TESTING PROVIDES THE ROADMAP YOU NEED 19

Chapter 3   THE RISA GROUX NUTRITION DETOX PLAN 33

PART II THE FOODFRAME EATING LIFESTYLE 65

Chapter 4   THE PALEO FOODFRAME 69

Chapter 5   THE KETOGENIC (KETO) FOODFRAME 87

Chapter 6   THE AUTOIMMUNE PROTOCOL FOODFRAME 111

Chapter 7   THE VEGAN FOODFRAME 135

Chapter 8   THE LOW LECTIN FOODFRAME 161

Chapter 9   THE LOW FODMAP FOODFRAME 181

Chapter 10   LIFE BEYOND THE FOODFRAME 207

APPENDIX I   RISA GROUX NUTRITION SUPPLEMENTS 211

APPENDIX II   MOST COMMONLY ORDERED TESTS 215

INTRODUCTION
How Hashimoto's Changed My Life

Jim Germanakos was the Season 4 champion on *The Biggest Loser* in 2007. He lost an astonishing 186 pounds on the show.

Within less than two years he gained it all back. And more.

Why did that happen? Why did most of the other contestants during that season--and every other season--gain all their weight back, and then some?

More importantly…why do *you* gain weight as soon as you stop dieting? Why don't diets ever work for *you*?

I think it's safe to say that we've all been on some type of diet in our lifetime. A diet touted by a friend, a relative, or a random celebrity. A diet they swore was the answer to your weight-loss and wellness needs.

A diet that you tried…but which failed to provide any long-term positive result.

And you know what? *It wasn't your fault.*

Let's be honest…diets don't work! Or rather, many may work in the short term, but they are intended to achieve one goal and one goal only: weight loss. That is old-fashioned and narrow-minded thinking!

Don't get me wrong, I am all for weight loss, but I firmly believe that it is a side effect of wellness. With the wide range of reversible diseases, we're dealing with, isn't it time to focus on wellness?

If there were a one-size-fits-all diet, you wouldn't be reading this book! And my job would be a lot easier, as I'd be able to put all my clients on an identical program.

As a functional nutritionist, I've treated thousands of clients over the last ten years, I know my system works. I call myself a wellness hunter because I focus on wellness and its foundational issues: systemic inflammation and gut health.

I know why the diets you've tried haven't worked. The reason is that each needs to be customized to your needs.

Research published in *Obesity Reviews* [1] in December 2018 looked at the diets, habits, and physical activity levels of hundreds of modern hunter-gatherer groups and small-scale societies whose lifestyles are like those of ancient populations. They found that *"they all exhibit generally excellent metabolic health while consuming a wide range of diets."*

Several high-profile experts, including Herman Pontzer, an associate professor of evolutionary anthropology at Duke University, and Michael Gurven, an anthropologist at the University of California-Santa Barbara, confirmed there is no one "true" diet for humans. Instead, *"they can be very healthy on a wide range of diets."*[2] That's because you have a unique history, genetics, gut microbiome, toxin exposure, virus load, disease profile, and lifestyle--so why would someone else's diet be right for you? Let me add that when I use the word "diet," I'm referring to an eating plan or lifestyle. This book will tell you exactly how to find the right one for you.

Even better, I'll tell you exactly what to eat. And what *not* to eat.

Although bookstore shelves are overloaded with diet books, most people simply do not know what to eat. Or how much to eat. They're given contradictory advice by their doctors--who most probably only received a few hours of instruction in nutrition, the media, their friends, and their family. This is one of the reasons why it's been estimated that 70 percent of Americans are overweight or obese. Childhood obesity has *tripled* in the last 30 years; one out of three American children is overweight or obese. One out of every child born today will become a type 2 diabetic. These are terrifying figures!

---

[1] https://www.nytimes.com/2018/12/18/well/eat/is-there-an-optimal-diet-for-humans.html
[2] https://www.nytimes.com/2018/12/18/well/eat/is-there-an-optimal-diet-for-humans.html

So, when Jim Germanakos came to me in despair, I instantly knew what *he* was doing wrong. When he'd been on the show, the focus had been extreme calorie restriction coupled with excessive exercise that no one except professional athletes could possibly continue once outside the confines of a reality show. He hadn't been given any help whatsoever with transitioning from such a controlled environment to eating in the real world—all he knew was how to count calories. He was putting a whopping nine packets of artificial sweeteners in his coffee each day, thinking this was better than sugar because they have no calories, and was shocked when I told him how bad this was. Not just for his health but as a hindrance to weight loss, as researchers have recently found that one common artificial sweetener, sucralose, increases the chances of glucose intolerance and other metabolic conditions that can result in higher blood sugar levels and a heightened risk of obesity.

So, what finally worked for Jim? I immediately put him on my 28-day detox plan and told him to eat when he was hungry and not to eat when he wasn't. To eat only real food and nothing packaged, processed, or artificial. Every day, he made two protein shakes and enjoyed one to two meals, with an optional snack if needed. We also set up an exercise plan to move his body by doing something he enjoyed. He worked out four to six times per week, but not excessively as he'd done on the show—he needed to learn how satisfying it is to have a sustainable, fun routine.

It only took those 28 days for Jim to lose 27 pounds. He hadn't been hungry or tempted to binge. He found it incredibly easy to stick to the plan. His energy skyrocketed and his joint pain disappeared. He went on to follow the Paleo diet you can read about in Chapter 3 and continued to lose weight and optimize his health. He was so grateful that he'd finally found the answers to his dieting dilemmas.

Now, you can too!

I genuinely believe that it's much more important to go after the root cause rather than treat the symptoms if someone is not feeling well or when the testing I do with them indicates that something is not quite right. I have witnessed incredible changes in people's health and in many cases, a complete reversal of autoimmune symptoms.

And, of course, these people have also lost an incredible amount of weight.

One of These FoodFrames Will Be Right for You

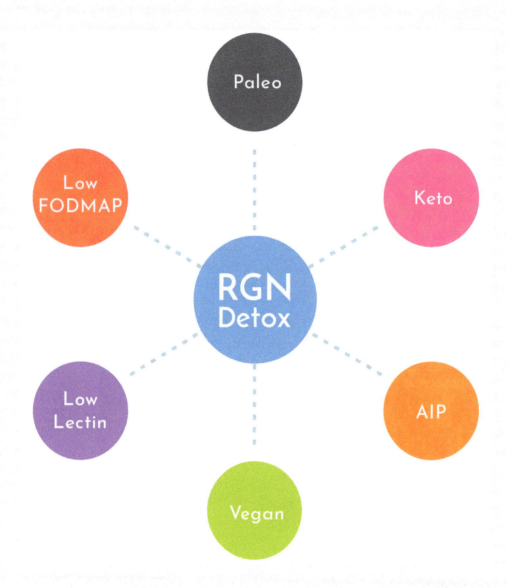

People walk in my office daily, confused about what to eat. They are spending all their energy on trying to lose weight, but losing weight is a side effect of *wellness*. We all need to look at the root causes and eat to address them and heal them.

This book will show you how to assess what's best for *you*. First, you'll do this with my FoodFrame quiz that you'll find online at www.Risagrouxnutrition.com and through assessing your health status. This will lead you to the FoodFrame that's the best eating lifestyle for your needs. Bear in mind that the RGN Detox is the recommended starter for every plan, so you should always begin there. The plans include:

- The RGN Detox
- Paleo
- Ketogenic
- Autoimmune Protocol
- Vegan
- Low Lectin
- Low FODMAP

HOW THIS BOOK CAME TO BE

I wrote this book for you, your loved ones, and your friends and colleagues who need as much information as they can get about how and what to eat. I know what it feels like to live without answers about your health concerns and to be confused about how to approach them. I personally know the deep and real frustration of doing all the right things and not seeing the weight loss results that have been earned.

I wrote this book because I don't want people to try every diet or diet type on the planet before they find their best fit. This book had to be written because I see people each day suffering from exhaustion and frustration on their health journey, and who are desperate for individual guidance. There are only so many people I can personally see in my office, and I feel that all of humanity is entitled to this information!

My parents were foodies before the word was coined. As a child I lived in Los Angeles and New York and loved to cook. I grew up loving to eat, and by the time I was a teenager I was eagerly trying every fad diet that announced itself as the best new thing. My weight was perfectly normal but, like most kids my age, I always thought I was fat. I yo-yoed from weight loss to weight gain, passed out from sugar imbalance, and got so tired at times that I could barely put my leg warmers on and make it to my step class.

As I grew older, I realized that my passion for food wasn't just the fun of concocting new recipes but the inextricable connection between food and wellness. Thankfully, I had come to learn that fad diets were merely short-term solutions to long-term symptoms. (Diets don't address why you got/get fat--they simply address the solution, not the root cause). And my years of expertise in marketing led me to understand the hype behind many diet claims, which often negated the science for an erroneous and often health-threatening hard-sell.

Like most diet-conscious Americans, I ate a typical diet of grains and low-fat foods. Fat was the enemy. When I was ready to start a family, I quickly received the good news. I had a healthy pregnancy and delivery of my daughter Sarah. A few years later, we were ready for me to get pregnant again, but after a year and a half of failed attempts, it was clear something was wrong. I went to a fertility specialist in despair, and after a battery of blood tests, my doctor told me I was hypothyroid--my thyroid gland function was abnormally low, and that could impede my ability to conceive. He handed me a prescription for Synthroid, a synthetic thyroid medication, and told me to take one every morning.

"How long will I need these for?" I asked.

"Oh, forever," he replied.

That is the moment when my journey to holistic wellness began. Why hadn't my doctor been curious about the *why* of my dysfunctional thyroid? Why did he tell me to just take a pill for the rest of my life without explaining all the potential pros and cons? Why didn't he want to fix the *root cause*?

This was not good enough for me. I started researching thyroid disorders as soon as I got home. I did not want to rely on something foreign to replace a function that my body was designed to do--I wanted to fix it rather than throw a pill at it. So, I went to see other experts. I tried acupuncture, herbs, Neuro Emotional Technique (NET), exercises, meditation--anything holistic to heal my thyroid and help me get pregnant. Finally, I went to see a highly recommended authentic Japanese acupuncturist whose office was sandwiched between a laundromat and pawnshop in a rundown part of town about a 30 minute-drive from home. He barely spoke English, so I pointed to my belly and said, "Baby" and he nodded his head. "Come 10 times," he said, and after seven visits, I had a positive pregnancy test, and a lovely, easy, complication-free pregnancy.

After my son Chase was born, however, I started exhibiting symptoms of thyroid issues again. I was tired all the time, couldn't seem to lose weight efficiently, my hair was thinning, and my nails were brittle. I didn't want to be dismissed or handed a prescription for a lifelong medication again, so I consulted a naturopathic doctor. After she tested my thyroid antibodies, I was told I had Hashimoto's Thyroiditis, an autoimmune disease in which antibodies directed against the thyroid gland lead to chronic inflammation. It is the most common cause of hypothyroidism in the US, affecting one in 34 people. Most of them are women over the age of 35-40, but it can also appear at any age, in men, and in children too.

My naturopath put me on WP Thyroid, a desiccated porcine thyroid hormone; I found out that all the natural ones are made from animal thyroid glands (usually a cow or pig). For me, it was a better choice than Synthroid. Not only was it natural as it was made from a living mammal, my body knew what to do with it, but it also contained both the T4 and T3 thyroid hormones I needed in higher doses. In contrast, Synthroid only contains a synthetic T4.

I became determined to find the root cause of my Hashimoto's so I could reverse it without *any* medications, synthetic or not. I completely removed gluten, dairy, and soy from my diet once my research showed me that gluten can trigger an immune response; the protein in dairy can also worsen autoimmune conditions; and soy can inhibit the thyroid's ability to absorb thyroid medication as well as iodine, which is essential for the production of the T3 and T4 thyroid hormones. I became a near-total vegan, eating plant proteins such as legumes, nuts, and seeds, and supplementing this with fresh fish or eggs every few weeks. I also reduced the number of high-impact workouts I'd been doing once I discovered that they could affect autoimmune disorders. I also had my heavy metals tested and was shocked to learn I had sky-high mercury levels, so I did a supervised chelation therapy for a year with great success.

My experience was one of the reasons why I decided to study for certification as a holistic nutritionist at this time. Through my research, I created a checklist of all the possible causes of Hashimoto's as I couldn't find root causes anywhere I looked. Not surprisingly, I tested positive for everything on the list. Even though I had been vegan for several years and ate an incredibly healthy diet, I was consuming so many plant-based carbohydrates each day that my blood sugar levels started rising without me eating any sugar at all! I continued to get my thyroid regularly checked and it was not getting better.

After years of searching, I finally found a doctor who understood autoimmune disorders. After even more extensive testing we determined that my blood sugar was dangerously high, in fact it was 0.10 % away from being pre-diabetic, along with elevated inflammation markers. I also did a specific heart health test and it showed that the marker for having a heart attack was twice the upper limit of normal. At that point, I knew something was still gravely wrong and took some action. I changed my diet from vegan and instantly removed legumes, grains, fruits, and nightshades from my diet and went on the Autoimmune Protocol Diet for 90 days. Since carbohydrates turn into sugar, I believed that my elevated glucose numbers were not due to my diet since I very rarely consumed natural sugars and never had processed sugar. I continued to eat 80 percent of my food from greens and vegetables but replaced the plant proteins with free-range, pasture-raised chicken and turkey along with wild-caught fish daily. I also took a boatload of supplements to address the cascade of inflammation and was 100 % compliant.

But after my 90-day re-check, the needle had only moved slightly, and the air was sucked out of my sails. While I was discouraged, I did not give up. I ordered myself a stool test and when it came back, the answer was staring me in the face. Not only did I have bacteria that can cause Hashimoto's in my gut, but I also had it in my saliva, which I was able to treat naturally with diet and supplements. At that point I began to make the connection between blood sugar dysregulation, or dysglycemia, and systemic inflammation. Dysglycemia occurs when there is an imbalance of either low blood sugar referred to as hypoglycemia or elevated blood sugar, known as hyperglycemia. Systemic inflammation happens when the body experiences chronic activation of the immune system as a result of lingering attacks to the body either from an autoimmune or chronic issue that creates an immune response. This, coupled with extremely elevated serum cholesterol levels, led me to my next step.

I knew oral health and heart health are related, so I quickly made an appointment with a holistic periodontist in Beverly Hills who took one look at my test and sent me straight to her MRI machine. Within minutes we saw it. An abscess had grown around a wisdom tooth root which remained after my wisdom teeth had been extracted 23 years earlier. It settled in my jaw- bone with absolutely no pain, swelling, tenderness, or symptoms of any kind. A few weeks later, I had surgery to remove the abscess and the root, while continuing to eat a Paleo diet. My blood sugar and thyroid started to normalize.

I believe the abscess had developed because of a bacterial infection which I discovered through my stool test. The chronic infection that existed for years caused systemic inflammation. Chronic, or systemic, inflammation suppresses insulin by signaling pathways to lower the body's responsiveness to insulin therefore increasing the likelihood of insulin resistance. In addition, long term inflammation can create oxidative stress in the body which affects thyroid function.

The stool test that gave me the answers I needed is the same test I order for just about every client, as it is a bit of a crystal ball. It tests for over 82 pathogens, fungi, parasites, and worms along with a lot of useful information regarding intestinal health.

A basic tenet of my practice is that if someone is not feeling well or their testing indicates something is not quite right, I go after the *why*. (Unlike my fertility doctor!) As I mentioned already, this is almost always due to systemic inflammation and/or gut health. If your body has one or both, chances are high that you will experience ill health. Intestinal permeability (or leaky gut), for example, can exhibit symptoms ranging from malabsorption, a depressed immune system, fatigue, headaches, diarrhea, constipation, gas, bloating, allergies, headaches, joint pain, and cravings.

This is why I use many tools in my practice to assess a person's health--I'm a big fan of playing darts with all the lights on so I can clearly see the target I'm aiming for! In addition to stool and blood testing, food allergy testing is also an important piece of the puzzle, as it's a safe assumption that you might have food sensitivities if your gut is compromised.

Every person has a unique physiology and genetic makeup and different exposure to toxins, diseases, and food, so everyone needs their own personalized eating lifestyle. *Food Frame* will teach you how to choose the best eating plan for your own health needs. These needs can change over time--and so should your diet type--which is it's good to always be in tune with your current state of health by routinely taking comprehensive blood tests and observing how your body communicates.

In this book, I chose the most common FoodFrames that I recommend for clients in my practice. I know how well they work because I see my clients' health improve and the pounds melt away.

You can easily work some of these ways of eating into your lifestyle, while others are elimination diets that help teach you how to listen to what your body tells you it needs. Each diet is a kick-start of sorts for a healthy, long-term lifestyle. One of the best things about the FoodFrame method is that when you know what to eat, you'll not only lose weight--because, as I've previously said, weight loss will always be a side effect of wellness--but you're going to feel so much better, have improved energy, stamina, better sleep, and mental clarity.

Just the other day, I asked a client how he was doing on his second week of the detox.

"My body is rejoicing," he told me.

It's time for you to rejoice, too! So, let's dive in and learn about the FoodFrame method that can promote optimal health and weight loss.

PART I

IMPROVE THE WAY YOU EAT

CHAPTER 1

GROUND-FLOOR ESSENTIALS FOR HEALTH WITH EVERY EATING LIFESTYLE

I wish there were a magic pill that could give us all our optimal weight and wellness. But there isn't. But you probably know that true health comes from every decision we make every time we put food and drink into our mouth.

When all new clients come to see me, I always tell them this: "I want you to imagine that your body is just like a sneaker factory. You have all the equipment you need to make a sneaker. If I give you rubber, leather, or canvas I know we will get a sneaker at the end of the line; it might be in different sizes, shapes, styles, or colors, but we would still get a sneaker. But what if I tell you I have a brilliant idea to put cellphone parts in your sneaker factory. What would you say?"

At that point, my new clients look at me with some degree of confusion, and, usually, they tell me, "I'd say, 'That is a really dumb idea'!"

"Yes, of course it is!" I reply. "Because you don't have equipment to make cellphones; you have equipment to make sneakers. The cellphone parts would break all the sneaker-making machines. So, I want you to think about how we humans have a body that's designed to eat nourishing food (our sneaker materials) for our bodies (the sneaker machines) to function optimally and efficiently. When we were created, there were animals crawling on the ground and foods sprouting from the earth that we could eat to sustain us and give us the ability to procreate, which are the two main basic functions of the human species. Then the industrial revolution came, chemical compounds were invented and used in abundant and increasing levels. That is when modern diseases became prevalent. If we continually put junk food and chemicals in our bodies, we can easily predict that our body systems and functions will begin to breakdown. Just like the cellphone parts would break the sneaker machines. Real food is the way to go! It is what we were designed to eat."

Fortunately, all the diets in this book are about eating real food. These are not fads or trendy "diets" intended for short-term success. They are long-term eating lifestyles intended for a lifetime of ultimate health benefits. They focus on eating for survival, in other words the focus is on eating foods that sustain, nourish, and heal rather than those with a lesser nutrient value eaten for pleasure, what I call eating for sport, such as sweets, processed foods, or alcohol. They will nourish and support the body for optimized wellness. Remember: Weight loss will be the result of that lifestyle.

So, I want you to use this chapter as a substitute for one of my personal consultations.

THE 4 FOODFRAME STEPS

Step 1 Take the FoodFrame Quiz

This quiz will direct you to the right FoodFrame. I designed the quiz to zero in on which eating lifestyle or FoodFrame is the best fit for you. It is matched with your current health status so there are a few simple questions that will help make that determination.

The FoodFrame method achieves the goal of decreasing inflammation and increasing good gut health, but it's not one size fits all. For example, some people can eat nightshades regularly while others cannot. Some can enjoy onions and garlic while these foods could damage the gut of others. It is imperative to know what heals and hinders you and your body. Your health status may improve, or you may develop another condition or autoimmune disease as a result of not addressing the root causes which may bring on an additional diagnosis. This is why I invite you to retake the test to determine if the changes are going in the right direction. Our bodies are always changing and it's essential that our nutrition needs accommodate those changes.

Simply go to my website, www.Risagrouxnutrition.com, and you'll see the quiz on the homepage. It's only 12 questions long. What are you waiting for?!

Step 2 Do the RGN Detox

You'll see exactly what to do in Chapter 3.

Step 3 Eat According to Your FoodFrame Type

The different FoodFrames are found in chapters 4-9.

Step 4 Accelerate the Results with Supplements

The information you need is in each of the chapters in Part II.

BEFORE YOU START

Now that you know which FoodFrame is best for you right now, there are two things to do:

- Read this section, as the basic guidelines apply to everyone and every diet type. They are the pillars of health and imperative for long-term success. Go at your own pace to achieve a comfortable

level of compliance. Some people can jump in with both feet right away, and others need to slowly stair-step it, so do what's best for you.
- Get the testing you need done. Go to Chapter 2 for guidance, as it will give you detailed information about all the tests that might be right for your needs. It is critical to look under the hood so you can clearly see the target. Let's find out what the root issues are if there are any to address. You can certainly start the process while you are waiting for test results, don't let that stop you.

1. **Exercise Does a Body Good**

We all know that moving our bodies on a regular basis is something we should be doing. Exercise will not just help increase your metabolism and therefore your weight loss, but it has many other benefits:

- Boosts the immune system
- Builds and maintains strong muscles and bones
- Helps brain health and memory
- Increases lifespan
- Increases weight loss
- Improves mood; decreases anxiety and depression
- Improves sex life
- Improves skin health
- Improves sleep
- Increases circulation and oxygenates the blood
- Increases energy
- Reduces chronic pain
- Reduces cortisol
- Reduces heart disease
- Stabilizes blood sugar

What you eat and drink is 70-80 percent of the weight equation. The remainder are exercise and lifestyle. Whether you hula-hoop in your underwear at home, walk the stairs at work, go to the gym, dance in the kitchen, practice yoga or Pilates, swim, take the dog for long walks, lift weights, jump rope, or run marathons...just pick something that you enjoy and do it often. You'll never want to exercise if you don't love doing it.

Remember: Abs are made in the kitchen. Six-packs are made in the gym!

2. **Color Your World with Vegetables**

When humans were first created, there were creatures crawling on the ground and plants sprouting from the earth--plants we could eat to survive and procreate, our two main living goals as human organisms. Then the industrial revolution came and created chemicals which have become increasingly prevalent in our daily lives. The widespread use of toxic chemicals has paralleled the increasing rates of disease. Now, nearly everything we breathe, consume, and place on our skin is affected in some way by these chemicals. Even organic foods show trace amounts of toxic chemicals, specifically glyphosate, the main ingredient in the herbicide, RoundUp.

Despite this, you still need your veggies, and you need them every day. Not just for their nutrients, but for their fiber. Most Americans do not eat enough high-fiber foods. I call fiber the waste train because it is not digestible; its sole purpose is to go through your digestive system and pick up or cling to waste (toxins or unusable particles) that don't serve in nourishing or supporting the body. You take your garbage out of your house regularly, right? Same thing applies to fiber, it helps eliminate the waste from your body.

In addition to escorting out the unwanted and unnecessary, fiber has many health benefits such as fighting against cancer and cardiovascular disease, lowering cholesterol; regulating blood sugar levels and obesity, reducing the risk of developing kidney stones, bowel regularity, and helping your body develop and maintain a diversified microbiome that aids in the processing of blood sugar. There is absolutely no fiber in animal protein or fats, which is why it's imperative to get it from its most abundant source: plants.

All but one diet type in this book contains unlimited vegetables. My belief is that 60-80% of your plate should be vegetables at every meal. This works out to four to six servings per day. These veggies can be raw, steamed, stir-fried, air-fried, roasted, grilled, baked, or put into a smoothie. Any way you want them but not but not deep-fried.

Vegetables all contain an abundance of nutrients, including vitamins and minerals, that you can't get from other foods. I always suggest you eat a wide array of colors as they all have unique health benefits and properties.

Another wonderful result of eating vegetables that are high in fiber is that this creates satiety. All that fiber will help keep you full and fueled.

SIDEBAR – How Much Fiber Do You Need?

- For adults ages 18 and up, I recommend 25 grams of fiber for women and 38 grams for men per day.
- For toddlers: 19 grams daily.
- For kids 4-8 years old: 25 grams daily.
- For girls 9 and older: 25 grams daily.
- For boys 9 and older: 31-38 grams daily.

As for calories, I am not a big believer in counting them as I would rather see you focusing on the *quality* of food. All calories are not created equally. If you have a budget of 1,200 calories in a day, does that mean you can eat ice cream and cookies to meet that number? Of course not!

I passionately believe in eating the nutrient-dense foods our bodies were built to process. When you eat quality food that nourishes your body, you will not require as much food as when consuming empty-calorie, nutrient-void foods. But for those of you that are focused on calories, another asset in vegetables is their low-calorie content. For example, one cup of cooked broccoli has 30 calories and 2.2 grams of fiber; one bowl of cooked white rice has 204 calories and 0.6 grams of fiber. One cup of almonds contains 12.5 grams, and one ounce of chia seeds contain 10.6 grams of fiber.

Vegetables also contain a fair amount of protein. It is important to remember that we need protein every day to build muscle, hair, nails, hormones, enzymes, neurotransmitters, and to repair tissue. The typical American diet overestimates actual protein needs—it's a lot less than you think! And eating too much protein can be a strain on the kidneys, especially for someone with a history of impaired kidney function. Overconsumption can also cause constipation.

SIDEBAR – How Much Protein Do You Need?

Protein requirements vary depending on weight, age, level of activity, and gender. If you are an athlete or work out heavily, you will need more protein. My rule of thumb for the professional athletes I work with is 0.7-1.0 ounces of protein for every pound they weigh, but the numbers vary from individual to individual, so check with a practitioner or trainer to see what's best for you.

The RDA (Recommended Daily Allowance) by the US government is 0.36 ounces per pound of body weight for non-athletes. Just multiply your weight by 0.36 to calculate your protein RDA.

3. **Drink Up—Water, That Is!**

Without water, we would die. We wouldn't die, however, without coffee, soda, iced tea, Frappuccino, or energy drinks…just without plain old water. Hydration is critical for brain function and energy production, prevention of headaches, regular bowel movements, to prevent kidney stones, induce weight loss, maximize physical performance, regulate skin health, for joint lubrication, saliva, and mucus production, to oxygenate the body, regulate body temperature, maintain blood pressure, and to optimize mineral and nutrient absorption throughout the body.

Adult humans are roughly made up of 60 percent water, but most of us don't drink anywhere near enough. I recommend half your body weight in ounces of water each day. For example, if you weigh 160 pounds, you should consume 80 ounces of water daily, or close to it.

What type of water is the bigger question. Unfortunately, the tap water in the United States is not always the cleanest source as it can be laced with chemicals and hazardous contaminants like disinfection byproducts, traces of pharmaceutical drugs, and fluoride. Most plastic water bottles contain BPAs (bisphenol A) and BPSs (bisphenol S), resulting in endocrine-disrupting chemicals, especially those that mimic estrogen, these can over time cause damage. (And not just to your body, but also to the environment.)

If you need to buy bottled water, I recommend spring water as it is the cleanest form available. (Make sure the brand you choose is actually real spring water, as some companies make untruthful claims about the source.) Filtered water is a slight step up from tap water but has miles to go to be considered pure water. Glass, porcelain, or stainless-steel bottles are always preferred over plastic, even if it's BPA-free.

I also recommend installing a reverse-osmosis water system in your home, which can remove up to 99 percent of contaminants. You should have your water tested, as well. Check with your county health department; they should be able to help you for free or you can find a state-certified laboratory by calling the Safe Drinking Water Hotline at 800-426-4791 or visiting *www.epa.gov/safewater/labs*. This is especially important if you are pregnant, nursing, have young children, or if anyone in your household has a chronic illness.

Many of my clients ask me about alkaline water, and I tell them that it's a slightly controversial topic as there are those who believe wholeheartedly that it can reverse disease and aid digestion. Alkaline water helps to decrease the acid in the stomach, which is an excellent health goal for someone who knows for sure they have an acidic stomach, but what about the person who tends to be more alkalized, or is taking antacids or proton-pump inhibitors (stomach acid reducers) such as Nexium or Prilosec? Further alkalizing would impair that stomach. We need an acidic stomach to break down our food, and you can easily check your acid/alkaline levels with saliva pH strips that can be purchased at a pharmacy or online. I have yet to meet anyone who chew their food the recommended 20-35 bites before swallowing, so it's up to your stomach to do the job effectively. For the stomach to process the food well it must be acidic Without enough acid, you'll get some form of indigestion such as heartburn or acid reflux. Over time that causes plenty of destruction. We ideally want our stomach acidic and our blood alkalized.

Sparkling water is also in abundant supply these days. I enjoy a San Pellegrino several times a week; unlike Perrier, which is naturally carbonated, it gets its bubbles from carbon dioxide. (You can make your own carbonated water at home with countertop machines.) Unflavored sparkling water has no calories, but flavored sparkling water can have as many as a soda. It's not a health drink. Many of these cans or bottles contain artificial flavorings and sweeteners which can deter your goal of wellness and weight loss. Read the labels and look for clean and natural ingredients. Cans and bottles can contain toxins such as BPAs and PVCs which can cause ill health and obesity.

Some reports claim that too much carbonated water can impair digestive enzyme production, and it can certainly cause bloating from the gas if you consume large quantities of it, so I recommend drinking it in moderation. Water can be flavored with slices of lemon, lime, or orange; herbs like rosemary or mint; or veggies like cucumber. The delicious taste will encourage you to drink more.

4. **Sugar Is the Devil**

Sarah was my first-born and Chase arrived six years later. I made all their baby food from organic and natural ingredients and provided a wide range of flavors so their palates would be far more expansive than the usual bland stuff given to little ones. It was always so interesting for me to see what they liked or disliked, and to observe their relationship with those foods as they grew. Now as adults, they know what foods work for them and continue to thrive physically and mentally from nourishing whole food. As toddlers, when I took them to the grocery store, I would go straight to the produce section and grab a string bean or two or a vegetable or fruit that was being sampled that day. We passed on the cookies, other sweet treats, or fried chicken fingers that were frequently offered. Yes, my kids were exposed to sugar, but it was only occasionally, and it was considered a treat. It was not offered as a bribe or withheld as punishment. It was not something they had or expected to have daily.

Why am I sharing this here? Because I knew back when my kids depended on me for all their food that sugar is the devil, plain and simple. And, hard as it may be to believe, if you cut down on your sugar consumption, you honestly do lose your sweet tooth.

This is something most Americans really, *really* need to work on. In the 1800s the average American consumption was negligible at two pounds per year. In the 1970s the average American consumption rose to 123 pounds of sugar per year. In recent years, the average consumption has been 152 pounds per year. That's equal to six cups of sugar in one week! That is a shockingly unacceptable number.

No wonder the rates of type 2 diabetes are skyrocketing. No wonder people are in a state of systemic inflammation. No wonder people can't lose weight.

When you have blood sugar dysregulation, there will likely be a wide range of consequences, such as difficulty losing weight, thyroid dysregulation, adrenal dysregulation, inflammation, and low immunity. I test four markers for blood sugar with just about every client who walks through my door, as this information is critical in evaluating a person's overall health. You can see the specifics in chapter 2.

As health concerns and obesity rates soar in this country, it's long overdue to admit that our obsession with and addiction to sugar has to stop. It's an epidemic that needs attention on a national level, for every American.

Why Sugar Is the Devil

Whenever we eat sugar, the pancreas pumps out insulin to manage it. That insulin finds the newly ingested sugar and converts it into glycogen, which is then sent to the brain and every cell in the body to be used as energy. That is the fuel that keeps us alive.

But there's one big problem with this totally normal metabolic function. [Illustration Blood Sugar] Whenever you ingest more sugar or carbohydrates, which turn into sugar, than you need, the excess glycogen that's produced needs to be stored somehow, somewhere—that's a leftover trait from our earliest ancestors, when humans usually suffered feast or famine and needed to have access to calories during times of famine. This excess of glycogen is stored as *fat* in case we may need to access it later. Think of when you fill your car with gas, any excess can't be utilized, it just spills out. And, if the glucose receptors on your cells are closed or impaired from insulin resistance, your body will store that glycogen as fat. In other words, if the glycogen cannot penetrate the cell because of the damaged receptors, it has no choice but to park it elsewhere--into fat cells and fat tissues. It's a very efficient and effective way to gain weight.

Therefore, sugar makes us fat.

Sugar = fat isn't just about white table sugar (sucrose) or your kids' leftover Halloween candy. It's about any food, especially carbohydrates, that necessitates an insulin release to help with the process of metabolizing this food. Whenever you eat carbs, your body converts them into glycogen. Insulin, the hormone secreted from the pancreas, monitors your blood glucose levels and escorts the glycogen into your cells.

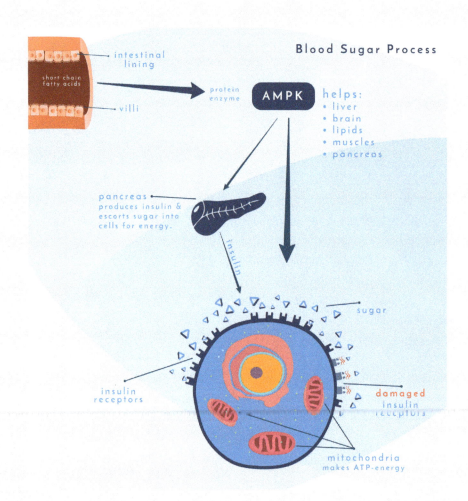

So, while we need a certain amount of carbohydrates for fuel every day, we need less than most people eat or that our government's food pyramid suggests. Potatoes, rice, bread, pasta, cereal, and pastries are all high-carbohydrate, high-sugar foods. Processed foods tend to be high in carbohydrates and low in fiber, which compounds the problem. All-natural sugars such as honey, maple syrup, or molasses are still sugar and they all create the same insulin/glycogen response. Fruit is another source of sugar even though its sugar is in the form of fructose rather than sucrose; fructose is processed primarily through the liver, but it still prompts an insulin release and spikes blood sugar levels the same way it would if you ate it in the form of a Twinkie. The fiber in the fruit will aid with a slower sugar spike, but will elevate blood sugar levels, nonetheless. Clearly there are more health benefits from eating an apple or some honey versus a piece of chocolate cake, but chemically, they all virtually create the same insulin-dependent/excess sugar stored as a fat response. And it will make you fat if you eat too much.

Here are some of the other unsavory things sugar does to your body:

- Chronic sugar consumption creates a fatty liver when fat is stored in it. A healthy liver is imperative for your entire body to work effectively, so when it's detoxifying capabilities are hindered, there will be a slow breakdown of the whole system. This is called Non-Alcoholic Fatty Liver Disease, which could lead to other serious diseases.
- Sugar is an inflammatory food and helps perpetuate systemic inflammation when blood sugar levels are chronically elevated. This happens all over the body, including the brain, which is why some scientists are now referring to Alzheimer's disease as type 3 diabetes—their studies are showing that there is now a strong connection between long-term blood sugar elevation and Alzheimer's.
- Sugar increases the risk not just of cardiovascular disease but of death because sugar increases our cholesterol and triglycerides levels.
- Sugar is nutrition for cancer cells. It helps them grow. No matter what kind of sugar it is--white sugars, processed sugars like agave, brown sugars, even fake sugars in the form of artificial sweeteners--every single type will nourish cancer cells, which is the last thing you want if you are suffering from this disease!
- Sugar causes fatigue. When blood glucose levels are elevated, it makes the blood sludgy. This slows down your circulation, which then hinders the distribution of oxygen and nutrients that your cells require. When blood glucose levels are low, there is an insufficient amount of fuel for optimal cell function.
- Sugar is damaging to the skin causing acne, dryness, and other issues. This is because it's a dehydrating agent. In addition, sugar affects your skin's water-binding capacity, so it can lose its radiance.
- When we eat sugar, it can destroy up to 50 percent of our white blood cells. It does so by attacking invaders such as bacteria, viruses,

parasites, and fungi. These cells are our immune system fighters, and when levels are low, we become vulnerable to sickness and disease.
- Serotonin is our mood-stabilizing, "feel-good" hormone, and 90 percent of it is produced in the gut. When sugar eats the good gut bacteria found in our intestinal microbiome, the total flora levels decrease while allowing the bad bacteria to take over lowering serotonin production levels.

Doubtless I just killed your buzz about sugar consumption, but that doesn't mean you can consider using artificial, chemically produced sweeteners such as Splenda (sucralose), Equal (aspartame and acesulfame-k), Sweet n' Low (saccharine), or any other no-calorie artificial sweetener. They're just as bad as sugar—if not worse. Your body can't tell the difference between real sugar and fake sugar. It still pumps out insulin in response, which leads to the same blood sugar spikes and the same fat storage. Artificial sugars have also been linked with health concerns such as cancer, tumor production, sugar dysregulation, insulin resistance, weight gain, hair loss, migraines, dizziness, and mood disorders. It's time to toss them. They are extremely destructive and, in my opinion, should be banned.

Does this mean you should never have a cookie ever again? Of course not. The less you eat sugar, the more your palate adjusts—really! Just as it did for my children, as I mentioned earlier in this section. For them, sweet potatoes or bright red raspberries were like candy. As adults now, my daughter loves homemade Paleo cookies (you can find the recipe on my website https://www.risagrouxnutrition.com/recipe/paleo-chocolate-chip-cookies) sweetened with monk fruit, and my son still loves to dive into a bowl of berries.

Be aware of how much sugar is in the foods you eat, especially processed or boxed foods. Read the labels and you'll see how many grams of sugar are in each serving. Some of the FoodFrames in this book include sugars like honey, maple syrup, coconut sugar, molasses, stevia, and monk fruit, but they are derived from real foods and recommended only in moderation.

Sugar alcohols, also known as polyols, are natural sweeteners that taste like sugar with fewer calories and negative effects of regular sugar. Common sugar alcohols are erythritol, mannitol, sorbitol, xylitol, lactitol, maltitol, and isomaltose. They have a different chemical structure than sugar and are partially resistant to digestion, so they become a bit more like fiber in the system. These are acceptable in some of the diets in this book. They don't spike blood sugar as much and don't contain grams of sugar on a label, so we are starting to see more foods containing them. They are minimally processed but can cause gas and bloating in some people or if you consume a lot of them. I would recommend these on the permitted diet types in moderation. Several sugar alcohols are found naturally in fruits and berries along with vegetables such as asparagus, sweet potatoes, carrots, and cauliflower.

Stevia, monk fruit and allulose still contain carbohydrates, although very few, so again I recommend them in moderation to my clients and use them in my own cooking.

Stevia is a natural sugar that comes from the stevia leaf. It's low glycemic and won't spike blood sugar levels. Some brands are highly processed, so I always recommend going with a liquid or powdered form of straight stevia.

Monk fruit is my personal preference and I use it for baking. Called Luo Han Guo in Chinese, it is a small green gourd that isn't palatable to eat but can be made into a tea or its extract processed into a powder or liquid as a sweetener. Several brands blend it with erythritol, a sugar alcohol, into powder like white table sugar. It is perfectly safe to use, does not spike sugar levels, is low glycemic, and has no aftertaste.

Allulose is a newer one on the market that is derived from figs. It is also at the top of my list as it does not spike blood sugar levels, is minimally processed, and has no aftertaste or gastric side effects.

5. **Time to Dump the Processed Foods**

The definition of processed food is technically any food that has been altered from its original form. Some forms of processed food are gently processed, such as canned tomatoes, frozen vegetables, or an oil pressed from a fruit like olive or avocado. Others are highly processed, like instant noodles, candy bars, soda, deli meats, microwave popcorn, breakfast cereals, and frozen/microwavable meals. Additional preservatives, additives, sweeteners, and/or flavorings are usually needed to ensure the shelf life of these items. Processed foods usually are low on nutrients and high in carbohydrates, sugars, bad fats, and processed salt.

When we eat these foods, our bodies need to discern between what is actual real nutrition and what is a foreign chemical to the body. This process demands energy and resources; with frequency, it can cause a host of health issues from fatigue, indigestion, constipation and bloating, depression, blood sugar dysregulation, vitamin deficiencies, leaky gut, and other health risks and chronic diseases.

Good health does not include eating processed foods on a regular basis. Once in a blue moon won't hurt some people, but when you eat real whole food, your body likes it and works optimally. My car was built with a tank for gas as its fuel source. I have never tried putting shampoo in it instead. Maybe the meter would register as full, but it would trash my engine and necessitate a lot of expensive and time-consuming repairs. My car was built for gas, and gas alone, so that is what I put in the tank, even if it's expensive and inconvenient. It's the same principle with your body. It needs the best possible fuel for the best possible health.

None of the FoodFrames in this book include processed foods. As a functional nutritionist, I do not recommend them either. I see first-hand what consuming processed foods on a regular basis does to my clients, and to other people I know.

Processed foods are guaranteed to contribute to your toxic load. They're often inexpensive because they use inexpensive ingredients like rancid oils or the cheapest cuts of meats that are often filled with antibiotics and growth hormones. Their convenience is undeniable, but we need to get back into the kitchen and reconnect with our food and know exactly what's on our plates. You are not a science experiment! If you want optimal health, you need to earn it—you're worth it!

6. **Healthy Fats Do Not Make Us Fat!**

Healthy fats are our friends. Healthy fats do not make us fat. As you read earlier in this chapter, *sugar* makes us fat!

In the 1950s, a physiologist named Ancel Keys declared war on all fat. He stated that it increased our risk for heart disease and was the sole culprit in causing weight gain. At the time, there was ample evidence otherwise proving sugar to be the actual culprit, but the government (and, suspiciously, the sugar lobby) chose to side with Keys. The media campaign that followed has caused a significant derailment in the true search for health. As a result, the increase of sugar consumption paralleled with the rise in obesity--and we are at an all-time high for both.

Dr. Mark Hegsted, a Harvard scientist, was hired and paid by the sugar industry to collaborate with sugar executives. He later became the director of nutrition for the United States Department of Agriculture and helped draft the government's dietary guidelines in 1977. Dr. Hegsted's paid research impacted government's dietary recommendations which positioned sugar as empty calories only effecting dental carries and blaming fat as hazardous for heart disease.

These executives and scientists with the help of a prominent Madison Avenue agency, further perpetuated the concept that if fat was bad for our health then sugar consumption would rise per capita, which turned out to be true and significantly added to the sugar industry's profits. In parallel, consumption of carbohydrates and the rate of obesity began to rise together.

Around the same time in 1972, a British professor of nutrition, John Yudkin was educating the public about the dangers of sugar in his book Pure, White and Deadly. His whistle blowing regarding sugar was promptly followed by a barrage of bad publicity by those in the food industry and his research and reputation never recovered during his lifetime. It is only from more recent science that reveals Yudkin was correct in that sugar is a major contributor of heart disease and obesity. [3]

As of 2019, one out of every three children born in the United States today will become a type 2 diabetic in their lifetime. That is a horrific statistic, and it needs to change. But it won't as long as millions of Americans eat processed foods laden with junk fats like processed and refined vegetable oils. And when junk fat is removed from packaged foods, it's replaced with sugar! Foods labeled "Low Fat" or "Fat Free" tend

---

[3] https://www.nytimes.com/2016/09/13/well/eat/how-the-sugar-industry-shifted-blame-to-fat.html

to have high levels of sugar or artificial sweeteners because without fat, they won't taste good. Sugar fills the gap. They are a must to avoid.

Eating the right type of fat is critically important to our overall health. Our brain is comprised of about 50 percent fat, so it is critical we feed it the right form of fat to sustain health and maximum functioning.

The healthiest fats are saturated and monounsaturated fats. It is also critical to have a balance of Omega3 and Omega6 polyunsaturated fats. An excess of Omega6 fatty acids leads to inflammation and gut dysbiosis, or an imbalance of good and bad gut bacteria, while Omega3 fatty acids help reduce inflammation, modulate the immune system, and feed our good gut bacteria. Many of our important vitamins require fat to be absorbed, especially vitamins A, D, E, and K.

Healthy Fats

- Animal fats from grass-fed and finished meats
- Avocados and avocado oil
- Coconut and MCT oil
- Olives and extra virgin olive oil
- Omega3 fats from fish
- Nuts and seeds
- Pastured butter or ghee
- Pastured eggs, yolks and whites

Healthy Fat Benefits

- Aids absorption of calcium
- Aids absorption of vitamins A, D, E, K
- Increases satiety
- Lowers cholesterol levels
- Maintains health of hair and skin
- Optimal fuel for brain and heart
- Provides building blocks for cells and hormones

Bad Fats

- Margarine and shortening
- Trans fats: anything fried or hydrogenated
- Vegetable oils: soybean, canola, cottonseed, sunflower, corn, safflower, rice bran, refined palm, refined grapeseed

Removing fats altogether is gravely destructive to our wellness, fertility, and weight loss abilities. Every diet type in this book contains good quality fats as they are integral for wellness and weight loss. Fat is not the enemy, so make sure to enjoy good quality fats every day.

7. **Macronutrients and Micronutrients for Optimal Health**

Macronutrients are protein, fat, and carbohydrates. How much should you eat of each? All the diets in this book have either different ratios of macronutrients, or no quantitative guidelines at all. There are different recommendations of the suggested daily allowance depending on who is making the recommendations. I don't suggest anyone getting out their calculator at every meal, which is why I've provided so many recipes as guidelines. I believe that our bodies know what and how much they need. We just need to learn to listen to them. And start by eating nutrient-dense whole foods.

Micronutrients are vitamins and minerals. Vitamins are necessary for energy production, immune function, blood clotting, and other functions. Minerals play an important role in growth, bone health, fluid balance, and several other processes. When you eat nutrient-dense whole foods, you are automatically ingesting all the amazing micronutrients your body craves.

8. **Let's Talk About Poop!**

Have you ever noticed how a baby eats a meal and poops shortly thereafter? Their transit time is so quick because their intestinal lining is so new and clean that the food they eat is absorbed and eliminated efficiently. This certainly isn't the case for adults!

Many people ask me how many times a day should they have a bowel movement. A normal range is one to three times a day, but there's no one right answer because frequency varies for each individual, and it also depends on several other factors such as:

- Diet
- Exercise
- Gut health
- Hormonal fluctuations
- Hydration
- Medications
- SIBO (Small Intestinal Bacterial Overgrowth)
- Sleep patterns
- Thyroid
- Travel

A normal bowel movement should be easy to eliminate; long, smooth, and formed; S shaped; medium dark brown; and with a uniform texture. It should sink to the bottom of the toilet; if it floats, this indicates that there might be an issue with how you metabolize fats. It should also be easy to wipe, without needing much toilet paper.

If you didn't take your household trash out for a week, you know it would stink, and even grow mold and bacteria. Feces are your body's equivalent of that household trash; they're the waste matter that remains after the nutrients have been extracted from the food you ate. They contain water, fiber, bacteria, and toxins from additives, preservatives, dyes, and chemicals. They need to be evacuated daily via your intestinal tract and rectum and flushed to eternity!

But constipation—when you have difficulty going, do not go daily, or need assistance with going--is extremely common in this country, and it's a huge problem. With chronic constipation, those toxins remain in the intestines and continually get reabsorbed into the intestinal walls. When compounded over time, this can be a huge contribution to the development of disease. I see a huge connection between regular constipation and hypothyroidism and SIBO (small intestinal bacteria overgrowth).

You can get your bowels to eliminate regularly again once you address the root causes. In addition to testing and addressing those issues, I recommend several things to help alleviate any constipation:

- Start the day with hot/warm water with lots of fresh lemon juice. (If you're taking thyroid meds, take them first wait one hour before drinking your water)
- Magnesium, specifically magnesium citrate, at night before bed as it relaxes your bowels and pulls water into the intestines. The water helps soften and bulk up the stool, which alleviates constipation
- Take a quality probiotic. If SIBO is suspected, find one without a prebiotic
- Increase water consumption
- Increase fiber consumption, unless SIBO is suspected
- Take postbiotics in the form of Short Chain Fatty Acids (SCFA) as they help improve the diversity of your microbiome and assist with elimination. They also assist in making a protein enzyme called AMPK that supports brain, liver, muscle, pancreas, and lipid functions, thereby regulating sugar metabolism.

The FoodFrames in this book will assist in improving all stages of digestion and promote regularity. By removing sugar, processed foods, and harmful ingredients while including lots of fiber, hydration, nutrient-dense foods, and exercise, your elimination process should work more efficiently, and you can say goodbye to constipation for good.

If it doesn't improve, then look for the root cause; it's quite common to experience chronic constipation from certain medications, a low T3, and/or SIBO. It's there--you just have to find it. The testing you'll read about in the next chapter is there to help guide you.

9. **Weight Loss**

I talk a lot about weight loss being a side effect of wellness, which is confirmed through my daily work with clients. I personally haven't dieted in decades and enjoy a wonderful Paleo eating lifestyle while maintaining my weight. Getting regular blood labs is a part of my plan to provide the internal roadmap. Our relationship with weight is something I find differs for everyone, but I find the majority are perpetually concerned with the number on the scale. Instead of thinking of weight loss as overwhelming or mystifying, take a look at these five major factors instead.

Blood Sugar: As covered in the sugar section, there are two mechanisms to assess. Excess fuel (sugar) your body receives will be stored as fat, and these reserves will increase if there are damaged cell receptors. To lose weight, give your body less fuel so it has no choice but to pull it from storage. When I work with people who have challenges with weight loss, I set a goal of net carbohydrates that works best for them for optimal weight loss.

Thyroid: Free T3 is the star of the show as it signifies if your burning capacity is on simmer, medium, or high. I can't tell you how many people walk into my office with severe, well-deserved frustration that they are doing everything right and can't lose a single pound. The first thing I do is check their Free T3. Their furnace is usually on simmer at best.

Sex Hormones: If you have a sex hormone imbalance, it will impair or curtail your weight-loss efforts. This is especially true for women as hormones change not only daily but several times throughout your lifetime. This tends to be an issue from hormonal imbalances as well as menopause when hormones shift substantially.

Cortisol: If the stress hormone cortisol is imbalanced, it can not only impede weight loss but effectively help weight gain. This can be addressed, but it's best to be tested before throwing darts in the dark. It's important to know what the dysregulation looks like in order to find the remedy.

Toxins: Toxins are stored in fat tissues and fat cells, so removing them will assist in weight loss. They are constantly accumulating, so strive to get rid of them regularly.

10. Immunity, Build Your Army

There has never been a better time to discuss our immune system! At the time of this book's publication, we are fighting one of the deadliest viruses in our lifetime, COVID-19 and it couldn't be more abundantly clear how critical it is to build our immune system for ultimate protection. In fact, we are faced with disease and viruses all the time, however, a virus requires a microbiome to house and nourish it. If we don't provide a sustainable environment, a virus cannot exist and flourish. Therefore, it is imperative that you address what you can control such as the food you eat so you can decrease your inflammation and increase your gut health, your microbiome.

Seventy-five to eighty-five percent of our immune system is produced in our gut which essentially is where our defending army comes from. Providing a steady stream of gluten, sugar, dairy, processed foods, and alcohol will continue to knock down our soldiers. Drastically decreasing or eliminating sugar or foods that turn into sugar will significantly assist in stabilizing blood sugar levels. This will result in increased inflammation, which is where disease loves to live.

Chronic systemic inflammation is the underlying cause of chronic disease. Simply changing our food choices can have a tremendous impact on our health. If you are like most Americans who are affected by heart disease, diabetes, cancer, autoimmune disease, or any other chronic condition, I invite you to eat for survival and not for sport. Take the FoodFrame quiz and determine which eating lifestyle will help put the inflammation fire out and recruit and repopulate more soldiers for your army, your microbiome.

Weight loss is a side effect of wellness, but immunity is a side effect of a clean and nutrient dense eating lifestyle.

You are not helpless against disease, each one of us has the power to build our immunity and experience optimal health.

CHAPTER 2

TESTING PROVIDES THE ROADMAP YOU NEED

Functional nutrition is the practice of viewing every aspect of one's current and past health, diet, symptoms, and overall lifestyle while using comprehensive science-based testing such as blood and stool tests to give current and accurate information and pinpoint exactly what root issues could be causing the body to be out of balance.

Functional Medicine was founded by Dr. Jeffrey Bland in 1990 with his strong vision for a care model that is grounded in biological systems and informed by research. It considers how interrelated every part of the body is. This strategy is implemented by looking at root causes of health and aims to create homeostasis in the body to restore physiological function at the best of its capability.

With functional nutrition, symptoms are clues for diagnosing primary health concerns, whether they are related to diet, illnesses, medications, lifestyle factors, exposure to toxins, antibiotic use, or other factors whereas conventional healthcare commonly tends to suppress symptoms with medication rather than treat the root cause. Functional nutrition sees these as evidence for understanding the underlying issues within your body. In essence, functional nutrition and functional medicine address the soil and trunk of a tree (the roots) where conventional medicine focuses on the branches (the symptoms).

Functional nutrition, however, is not a one-size-fits-all eating lifestyle because we are all physiologically different and our health status tends to change so it's critical to customize your eating plan taking your unique specifications into account to prompt healing from the cellular level.

Functional

- Looks at root causes
- Looks at the body as an inter-connected system
- Treats the whole body with food, supplements, and lifestyle
- Focuses on prevention

Risa Groux, CN

Conventional

- Treats symptoms
- Has specialists for each body system
- Treats an ill with a pill
- Treats disease already present

Functional medicine and functional nutrition are approaches to health that view most symptoms and diseases as the result of an imbalance in the body. Any excess, such as blood sugar dysregulation, systemic inflammation, or any deficiency, like not enough healthy intestinal bacteria, create an environment that promotes the development of ill health. Using this system is fully supported by scientific evidence, such as blood work or stool tests that look for potential pathogens, fungi, or parasites. It has been proven that when imbalances are corrected, symptoms and diseases can improve, even disappear. Health issues are not a result of a deficiency in medication but is rather a *root cause* creating ill health or severe and possibly long-term imbalances. If these root causes, or foundational issues, are not discovered and addressed, the body will perpetuate ill health which is likely to cause inflammation.

Take cholesterol for example. We need it to build and maintain cells, produce hormones, and vitamin D with the aid of digestion, particularly that of fats. If your cholesterol is elevated, it is usually an indication that something is inflamed or out of balance, commonly the thyroid or blood sugar. I look for the root cause and aim to bring the cholesterol within range naturally. The ranges for total cholesterol had been 185-200 for many years, but recently it's been moved to 99-169. Functional medicine keeps the range at 185-200, as cholesterol is neither a golf score nor the enemy. My feeling is that this happened due to pressure from the pharmaceutical industry, as this lower range will make it easier to justify a prescription for a statin to lower cholesterol, but that is just a hypothesis.

The functional approach has slightly more narrow lab ranges as it looks for prevention of disease, whereas conventional medicine tends to assess with wider ranges--which means they treat when disease becomes present, and not so much preventatively. In addition, all labs will adjust their ranges throughout the year.

These ranges are different for each lab company across the country. I tested this notion several years back when I took my son to two different labs in the exact same building about six weeks apart. I studied the ranges, and many were the same, but others varied from 0.10 to 400 depending on the marker. Labs tend to move to the median of what is coming in. For example, if they see a lot of hypothyroid, they will move the range to accommodate the average results--so you could be diagnosed with hypothyroid in Maine but not in Texas. In addition, labs are ordered with a heavy influence on what the insurance company will cover. Some companies do not cover many tests so the patient will glean very little information. I work with a few doctors who couldn't have their hospitals order the labs I requested as they stated that they didn't test those markers.

One of the biggest differences between my practice and that of most mainstream physicians and nutritionists is that I use a very specific testing regimen. I am a big fan of playing darts with all the lights on so I can clearly see the target. If the lights are dim, then I have to guess where the target is and won't be as accurate in my aim. This works amazingly well because these tests usually lead us to the root cause of health issues—but you won't know what these causes are unless you see the science behind them with the hard data from your test results. I've witnessed time and time again that once I can identify and address the *why*, my patients and I see a remarkable turnaround of the disease or health status.

Once I know exactly what is affecting your blood and your gastrointestinal tract, I can address it naturally. The two primary methods of testing are a comprehensive panel of blood work, to assess potential disease and imbalances that could lead to disease, and a stool test, to see what's going on in the gut that could be causing issues you might not be fully unaware of. If warranted, there are specialized tests for other conditions, but these two are the baseline tests I always begin with.

BLOOD SUGAR TESTING

The numbers are staggering. According to The Centers for Disease Control and Prevention, an estimated 30.2 million adults—12.2 percent of the adult population in the US— were living with diabetes in 2015, and 7.2 million (23.8 percent) of them were undiagnosed. An additional 84.1 million US adults are pre-diabetic, with nearly 90 percent of them unaware of their condition. What does this mean? Serious health complications on the horizon at a mind-numbing cost. According to the American Diabetes Association, the treatment of diagnosed diabetes in this country is a whopping $245 billion, *each* year.

Diabetes is a serious disease. It can lead to loss of limbs, blindness, systemic inflammation, leaving you with a compromised immune system, many other complications…and an early death. It is critical to find out if you have any kind of blood sugar dysregulation, not only for effective weight loss but to see if your numbers put you at risk for developing diabetes. This is one of the top two things I look at first because it affects so many functions in the body.

Type 1 diabetes is an autoimmune disease that attacks the beta cells in the pancreas and prevents the body from making enough or even any insulin; as a result, the body is flooded with blood sugar as it's difficult to enter the cells where it's needed. Type 2 diabetes is more common and is acquired mainly through diet— this means it can be reversed. It happens with insulin resistance and the body being unable to use insulin properly. The glucose cannot penetrate the cells; eventually insulin production stops; and the body is saturated with blood sugar.

The blood sugar tests I order are all done via the Comprehensive Bio Screen blood tests in a lab. I prefer that you ask for all four sugar markers listed below for a full evaluation. Once you have the results, you can determine if you have a blood sugar dysregulation issue (and other contributing factors). It is important to note that if you are concerned about your test results to seek out a functional practitioner to help interpret them or order further testing if needed. The four tests I request are:

Fasting Glucose. This test assesses your blood sugar levels at the time of draw, without you having eaten any food for 8-12 hours prior. This number can be affected by what you ate the previous day and can fluctuate a bit, which is why I don't rely just on this test as many practitioners do. Most labs and practitioners usually consider normal in the range of 80-100. Pre-diabetic levels are at 101-125. Anything exceeding 125 is considered diabetic. Functional ranges are 85-99.

Hemoglobin A1C. This test helps determine if you are within a normal range, prediabetic, or diabetic. Its number indicates what your blood sugar levels were over the previous three months. If this number rises significantly, I can see that my clients have likely developed significant insulin resistance and pancreatic beta-cell dysfunction. Functional medicine likes that number to ideally be 5.0-5.2. For reference, mainstream and functional medicine/nutrition agree 5.7-6.4 is pre-diabetic, and 6.5 and higher is officially diabetic. This range tends to move slowly so I recommend rechecking no less than three months apart.

Fasting Insulin. This test indicates the level of insulin circulating in your body while fasting. Your body needs insulin at all times, so you don't want it to be too low; too much, on the other hand, will indicate insulin resistance, pre-diabetes, or early-stage type 2 diabetes. In addition, high levels can lead to decreased levels of magnesium and HDL (good cholesterol), and elevated levels of LDL (bad cholesterol) along with inflammation. Too much insulin will promote weight gain by storing fat.

C Peptide. This test is the most stable marker of insulin and tells you how much of it your body is making. I use this test to determine if there is likely insulin resistance or diabetes. Insulin resistance is a precursor to type 2 diabetes. Both the mainstream and functional medical communities agree that anything 2.0 and above usually indicates insulin resistance or type 2 diabetes due to an overproduction of insulin. When it dips much below 1.5, it can indicate type 1 diabetes, as this is a sign that your body is not making enough insulin. I like that number to be 1.5 or close enough to it. This number will usually increase before the glucose is out of range so you can catch sugar dysregulation early. I rarely, if ever, see mainstream practitioners order this marker. It is extremely helpful, and I highly recommend getting it tested.

THYROID TESTING

Your thyroid is a small, butterfly-shaped gland located low on the front of the neck below the Adam's apple and in front of the windpipe. It is primarily responsible for regulating your metabolism, temperature gauge, and growth and development of your body, but it also affects a whole host of other bodily functions as well. This makes it critical to ensure that it is functioning optimally. I see so many people in my office with complaints of poor functioning thyroid, and their mainstream doctors have tested for it and told them they're at "normal" levels—and yet their symptoms continue because their doctors have repeatedly missed what's really going on. Some common symptoms of low-functioning thyroid, or hypothyroidism are:

- Brain fog
- Brittle nails
- Cold extremities (hands, feet, or generally running cold)
- Constipation
- Difficulty sleeping
- Fatigue, in many cases extreme
- Irregular menstrual cycles
- Memory issues
- Outer end of eyebrows missing
- Thinning hair
- Weight gain/inability to lose weight

Hyperthyroidism is when the thyroid is overproducing thyroid hormones. The symptoms can include:

- Difficulty sleeping
- Feeling nervous
- Hand tremors
- Heart palpitations
- Irregular menstrual cycles
- Irritability
- Mood swings
- Panic attacks
- Weakness
- Weight loss

Functional medicine typically looks at all 10 markers of the thyroid, as doing so will tell the whole story. Most conventional physicians will order only one to three at most, which always leaves me guessing as to what the root cause of my clients' thyroid issues are. When assessing the thyroid, I look for other hormones that may be affecting it—such as if the client is in a state of autoimmune disease where the body is attacking the thyroid falsely, thinking it's the enemy. As you know, I like to play darts with all the lights on so I can see the target clearly.

How Your Thyroid Works

When assessing the whole thyroid function, I look for several things involved in the process. Is there a production issue, a processing issue, conversion issue, and/or an immune response? You could have none, one, or all of those--but it's critical to see *all* the markers to determine what the issues are, if any. I look at thyroid hormones for free and total hormones. Free means it is unbound and available for usage. Total is the sum of what is free and what is bound to proteins. Both markers contain important information giving you the full story of how the thyroid is functioning and where it could be causing a disturbance. Thyroid function is quite complicated, it's easier to explain it with this list:

*Thyroid function begins with your pituitary, a pea-sized and shaped gland located in the center of your brain. The pituitary makes TSH, or thyroid stimulating hormone.

*TSH then goes through your liver, where it creates the T4 hormone. (This is why it's so important to detox, so your liver is always at its optimal functioning). T4 is your inactive thyroid hormone and makes up 93 percent of your thyroid hormones.

*That T4 needs to convert into the T3 hormone, which is the active thyroid hormone—but T3 is only seven percent of the equation! That's why, when I look at thyroid hormone levels, I always look at both the free and total numbers. Free means that it is unbound to any protein and available for usage, and total means the hormones that are bound to proteins combined with the free ones. The total numbers are helpful for guidance.

*The star of the show is free T3, the active thyroid hormone, a complex system of mechanics that leads to the production of free T3. Each step along the way needs to work optimally to obtain a robust free T3. Therefore, it is important to see each step, so I can then pinpoint where a breakdown may be occurring. The conversion process is critical in making T3, and selenium is an integral nutrient for proper conversion to take place. Decreasing levels of T3 indicate hypothyroid, meaning sluggish production of thyroid hormone. Hypothyroid is by far more common. Elevated levels of T3 indicate hyperthyroid, meaning an overproduction of thyroid hormone. To officially be diagnosed, your TSH result needs to be out of lab range. It's important to note that if you are on thyroid medication, the TSH tends to go very low as the pituitary does not need to work to make T4.

*The functional parameters are listed below, but it is important to note that if your free T3 is less than 3.0, this will usually indicate a difficult time with weight loss and promote most of the hypothyroid symptoms listed above. In addition, I look at Reverse T3, which essentially means that cortisol, one of your stress hormones made in the adrenal glands, is dysregulated, affecting, or bringing down your T3 levels. If I see this number is elevated, I address the adrenal glands and/or stress management.

*I also look at T3 Uptake, which indicates if estrogen (for a female) or testosterone (for a male) is competing for the thyroid cell site. If sex hormones are elevated, it will affect optimal thyroid function which is indicated in low level of T3 Uptake. In essence, this marker determines if the imbalance is binding excess estrogen or testosterone to thyroid hormones and impairing optimal thyroid function.

All those markers will give you a complete picture of what your thyroid hormone levels are, but I also want to see if your body is producing antibodies to its own thyroid gland. Antibodies are present when the body mistakenly targets components of the thyroid gland as the enemy and therefore perpetually attacks it. This is what happens when your body develops an autoimmune disease leading to chronic inflammation of the thyroid, potentially causing tissue damage and or and/or thyroid dysfunction. Unfortunately, I see this happen many times when my client's blood test results come in. The bad news is that there's a problem, but the good news is that I most likely found the source and can now address the root cause of the autoimmune disease. I look for two markers, Thyroid Peroxidase Antibodies (TPO) and Thyroglobulin Antibodies. If one or both are elevated and out of lab range, then antibodies are present in the blood. There are two types of autoimmune diseases related to the thyroid. Hashimoto's thyroiditis, an autoimmune disease with a hypothyroidism or underactive thyroid and Graves' disease, an autoimmune with a hyperthyroidism or overactive thyroid. To be diagnosed with one or the other, a person would need an abnormal or out of lab range TSH along with specific antibodies present. If you discover you have out of lab range TSH and high levels of antibodies, it is best to see your functional healthcare practitioner to take the necessary next steps for a clinical diagnosis. In the meantime, my advice is to follow the Autoimmune Protocol elimination diet for 30-90 days, as that should help with inflammation and symptoms.

Functional Optimal Thyroid Ranges for Adults

This testing is all done via blood tests in a lab.

TSH: 1.0-1.8 (unless on medication for T3 and/or T4 as that will usually lower this number)
Total T4 (Thyroxine): 8.0-8.9
Free T4 (Thyroxine): 1.5 or close to this number
Total T3 (Triiodothyronine): 130-150
Free T3 (Triiodothyronine): 3.5-4.0 is ideal but should be over 3.0
Reverse T3: 15 or just under is ideal, and 13-15 is best
T3 Uptake: 29 is ideal, but 27-30 is good too
Thyroid Peroxidase Antibodies (TPO) 0-10 is ideal but will take less than 34
Thyroglobulin Antibodies less than 1.0.

OTHER MARKERS

In addition to blood sugar and thyroid levels, I ask for other blood tests, as they will provide indicators to what might be out of range and perhaps which path to pursue. It is incredibly detailed to get into all the lab markers, but these are the key markers that I immediately look for and that would be helpful for you.

Vitamin D Markers

Vitamin D is critical for so many cellular functions of our foundational well-being that it's one of the markers I always look at first. Functional guidelines for Vitamin D 25 Hydroxy (D3) are 80-100. Those with autoimmune conditions can even go to 120 so it's best to request your D3 levels to be tested routinely.

Despite its name, vitamin D is not a vitamin, but a pro-hormone, or precursor of a hormone. Every cell in the body has a vitamin D receptor which affects gut, brain, heart health, and the nervous system. It is critical for immune support, thyroid, to regulate insulin, and cancer prevention. It is also necessary for strong bones. I don't care how much calcium you take or eat, as you will not make new bone without proper levels of synergizing vitamin D!

Unlike most other vitamins, it's challenging to get sufficient levels of vitamin D just from your food, so your body needs to manufacture it. You naturally make vitamin D after exposure to the sun—this needs to be for a minimum of 20 minutes per day without sunscreen or sunglasses. The darker your skin, the more challenging it is to absorb. The older the person, the harder it is to absorb as well.

The problem is that many people believe they have sufficient vitamin D levels, as they are outside for at least part of the day. In truth, most people are vitamin D deficient; even the professional athletes I work with who are outside almost all day, every day, tend to have low levels. This main reason being our soils which used to be rich in and was our main source of vitamin D is now depleted and cannot transmit it to the plants we eat because of the chemicals (pesticides, herbicides, glyphosate, etc.) used to treat it.

Signs of a severe deficiency are:

- Bone pain/loss
- Depression
- Fatigue
- Frequent colds/sickness
- Hair loss
- Lower back pain
- Muscle pain

A connection has begun to be made between the mortality rate of COVID-19 patients to low vitamin D levels. Think about the people at the highest risk of dying: people who are inflamed, overweight, or obese; those with darker skin tones; and the elderly living in nursing homes without much time in the sun. I said it earlier, but it bears repeating, vitamin D is critical for our immune system! Low vitamin D is a sign of inflammation, which, of course, you don't want.

Some foods like fatty fish, egg yolks, mushrooms, and liver contain vitamin D, but I recommend getting your levels checked and taking a quality vitamin D3 supplement. Look for one containing vitamin K as well, which assists in absorption. D3 is more absorbable than D2. In addition, most processed foods that are fortified contain D2 as it's cheaper. Make sure your supplements do not contain additives, colors, or oils, especially soybean oil, as they can quickly go rancid.

Inflammation Markers

I also initially test for two inflammation markers: homocysteine and C Reactive Protein (CRP). These can be cardiovascular-related and indicators of how much inflammation is in your body.

If homocysteine is elevated, it can prevent your body from naturally detoxifying heavy metals and toxins, so they will continue to be reabsorbed and cause inflammation. I like homocysteine to be around 6-7. We often see this elevated with the gene mutation MTHFR, which means the methylation pathways need to open to work efficiently. (See the MTHFR section on p. 43 to learn about methylation pathways, what they are and how they work.) CRP should be as low as possible; lower than 1.0 is ideal.

In addition, I look at liver markers ALT and AST, which I like to see in the teens or low twenties. If those levels are significantly elevated, meaning close to 50 or higher, there is most likely fatty liver or non-alcoholic fatty liver, and a detox would definitely be in order. If they are egregiously high, such as over 150, I would recommend seeing a physician, as this could be a sign of excessive alcohol or drug consumption, fatty liver, or viral hepatitis.

White blood cells (WBC), which fight off infections or illnesses, are also an important indicator of what is happening in your body. Functional medicine likes this number to ideally be around 5.0-6.0. If it's above 8.0, it will usually indicate that your body is actively engaging all its white blood cells to protect itself from an outside attack from a virus or bacteria. If the WBC is lower, perhaps lower than 3.0, then your body has been in a chronic state of inflammation or infection. Again, if your WBC is very out of range, seek prompt medical attention.

Iron Markers

Iron is the foundational element of all bloodwork. It's one of the most under-looked and critical components to the building blocks of health. A shortage or surplus of iron affects the body as everything is tied together to provide optimal health. An iron deficiency can throw off the thyroid and sugar markers.

When I look at iron, I primarily look for red blood cells (RBCs) first, as this is the initial indicator that there is a problem. If RBCs are low, anemia is likely to be present.

When your RBCs are starved of oxygen, basic functions to maintain, regenerate, or heal your body simply cannot operate optimally. RBC numbers can differ depending on your sex and where you live due to elevation, and B12, folate, thyroid autoimmune disorders, hormone imbalances, chronic illness, and medications can all cause the red blood cells to decrease.

I order the full iron panel, including TIBC (total iron binding capacity), iron saturation, ferritin, and soluble transferrin receptor, to get a full look. If the soluble transferrin receptor is high, iron is most likely needed. If low, iron supplementation is usually not needed and probably related to chronic illness. For iron saturation in males we aim for 40-50 percent, and in females 25-35 percent. Ferritin is your body's bank account for iron. Ideally, this number should be close to 100, but anywhere from 50-100 is acceptable. If iron is elevated, it could be from excessive wine or red meat consumption or using cast iron pans for cooking. Iron is tricky, so it's best to review your lab results with a functional practitioner.

If ferritin is extremely high, perhaps over 250, it is possible to have hemochromatosis, a condition where your body stores iron. This is more common for males but occurs in females, too, and usually appears around age 50, although it can occur anytime. Hemochromatosis can cause hormonal and other serious issues, and if unchecked can be fatal, so it needs to be promptly addressed with a medical professional. Some individuals can store iron without developing hemochromatosis it's also important to note that having high levels for a long period of time can be inflammatory.

MTHFR Gene Mutation Markers

If I find elevated homocysteine (a marker for inflammation) and/or MCV (the size of a red blood cell), it warrants testing for MTHFR (Methylenetetrahydrofolate reductase).

MTHFR is a quite common gene mutation found in 50-90 percent of the population, including me and my children. Because it is so prevalent, I ideally test every client I work with. It's common in those with thyroid issues. It is 100 percent hereditary, coming from either or both parents. If you have this gene mutation, you might have a hard time methylating either your B12 or folate (B9) or both. Methylation is a metabolic process that turns genes on and off and repairs DNA. It also affects nutrient conversions through enzyme interactions. Poor methylation can increase the risk for common disorders, as you'll see in the list below. MTHFR can also affect the way you metabolize and convert critical nutrients from your diet into minerals, vitamins, and proteins.

If you have the MTHFR gene, you can have high homocysteine levels and low levels of B12 and/or folate, but not everyone does. There are many symptoms; the major ones are:

- ADD, ADHD
- ASD (autism)
- Anxiety and depression
- Bipolar disorder
- Cognitive function issues
- Colon cancer
- Elevated cholesterol
- Fatigue
- Heart disease
- Infertility
- Migraines
- Miscarriages
- Nerve pain

If untreated, these can lead to inflammation, difficulty detoxifying toxins and heavy metals, and possible cardiovascular issues.

I recommend getting a MTHFR blood test for anyone with either a thyroid issue, an autoimmune condition, or any of the above symptoms. The solution is simple: Just take a daily methylated supplement specific to MTHFR, containing a methylated B12 and folate. It is equally important to avoid the synthetic form of folic acid as it can gum up your system and often worsen symptoms. Folic acid is found in multivitamins, processed flours, and breakfast cereals. Make sure to eat foods high in folate and B12, such as high-quality animal protein, asparagus, avocado, beans, brightly colored fruits, broccoli, leafy greens (especially spinach), and lentils.

Epstein-Barr Virus Testing

There are five types of white blood cells that all help attack invaders in your body. These cells are basically your army that stands guard and activates when necessary. If these three in particular--monocytes, neutrophils, and lymphocytes—are seen in elevated levels, it's an indication that testing for Epstein-Barr Virus or cytomegalovirus is necessary.

Epstein-Barr Virus (EBV) is one of the most common viruses in humans and can silently live in your body's cells for a lifetime. A member of the herpes virus family, it spreads mostly through bodily fluids, primarily saliva, although blood and semen are possibilities as well. Up to 95 percent of American adults have acquired the virus by the time they're 40, and about nine out of 10 adults will test positive for either active or latent EBV.

After you get EBV, the virus becomes dormant—but in some cases it can reactivate. (This is similar to what could happen if you had chicken pox as a child; the virus remains dormant but can reactivate in the form of shingles.) This might not always cause symptoms, but people with weakened immune systems are more likely to develop symptoms when reactivation happens. If you've had mononucleosis, you have EBV in your body, but the degree is unknown until tested. Typically, infectious mononucleosis usually appears 4-6 weeks after you're infected with EBV. Symptoms may occur slowly and not all occur at the same time.

In reality, while most people have EBV in their bodies, many have never developed mono or shown any symptoms of it. Although there is no current science that can prove the connection between autoimmunity and EBV, there are several theories linking them. It is known, however, that EBV-infected cells may turn on certain genes that cause autoimmune conditions, with the highest connection being lupus, multiple sclerosis (MS), chronic fatigue syndrome, fibromyalgia, Hashimoto's thyroiditis, and Grave's disease. EBV can be the root cause for up to 33 autoimmune diseases and dysregulate blood sugar and thyroid health.

If you guessed that I had EBV, you were right! I treated it with a supplement regimen that I still use with my clients to significantly decrease or put the virus in a dormant state.

Other Testing

If needed, I will order other blood tests based upon the initial results of the baseline testing. There are thousands of scenarios, so it's not possible for me to address them all in the confines of this book, but I do recommend that you seek out a functional healthcare practitioner. If something is awry, there is always a reason. Look deep and wide and don't give up!

STOOL TESTING

As you read earlier in the book, much to my surprise I learned that I had the bacteria that can cause Hashimoto's in my gut. This is only one of the reasons why stool testing has become an essential tool in my practice, as it is an expeditious and efficient vehicle in discovering root causes of health concerns such as:

- Anxiety, depression, and mood disorders
- Autoimmune diseases
- Blood in the stool

- Brain fog
- Diabetes and weight-loss issue
- Digestive complaints; constipation or diarrhea
- IBS/IBD
- Skin problems, such as acne and psoriasis

The correct microbial test done by a reputable lab can reveal pathogens such as bacteria, fungus, parasites, potential autoimmune triggers, viruses, worms, and yeast; and other intestinal health issues with markers including enzyme production, fat absorption, gluten sensitivity, immune function, inflammation in the digestive tract as well as antibiotic resistance.

I order a stool test with practically everyone I work with as it will give me tremendous information that is rarely looked at. I can't tell you how many times a person comes into my office with joint pain, and I find they have high levels of Prevotella Copri, a pathogen that can lead to rheumatoid arthritis. Bacterial infections such as Helicobacter Pylori (H-Pylori) or Yersinia, along with a parasite called Blastocystis hominis, have been associated with the root cause of Hashimoto's. There are countless pathogens that can trigger health issues and autoimmune disease and that is precisely why I look inside the intestines.

Extremely elevated levels of antigliadin IgA can also indicate the potential to develop celiac disease. A low secretory IgA will tell me about the level of immunity you have in your gut at the time of testing. Remember that 75-85 percent of our immune system is produced in our gut. So many of these pathogens can cause underlying chronic illness—but when properly addressed, can alleviate not just the symptoms but the high likelihood of developing the illness itself. Taking medicine for these issues is a Band-aid solution which can lead to other issues. It doesn't fix the problem. It is imperative to find the root causes!

Recently I tested what appeared to be a perfectly healthy 36-year-old man with no symptoms of any kind We found an elevated occult blood level, meaning blood in the stool that is not commonly visible to the naked eye. I urgently recommended he arrange for an immediate colonoscopy with his gastroenterologist and fortunately he heeded my advice. He had four large polyps and the biopsies showed they were cancerous. He had zero blood or mucus in his stool and absolutely no other indications that something could be wrong. Needless to say, his wife and two little girls were incredibly happy we looked under the hood.

Frequently, I have people come into my office who have only been stool-tested for a handful of bacteria--literally just four pathogens or yeast, which tested negative, and their doctor may have told them they are fine. If they're still frustrated with symptoms, I order blood work and a stool test. I use Diagnostic Solutions Labs, as they offer the most comprehensive qPCR test which screens for over 80 pathogens along with those I mentioned above. It even includes a section on antibiotic resistance because antibiotics are found consistently in our food and water. When you unknowingly ingest a steady stream of antibiotics, your body will eventually become resistant to them and will not work if needed at a time of crisis.

The GI MAP test kit is only available through practitioners, so it's best to find a functional medical professional who uses this test. After I see the results of the Comprehensive Bio Screen blood tests and the GI MAP stool tests, I will have the road map, the indicators, that will tell me if more specific follow-up tests are indicated.

CHAPTER 3

THE RISA GROUX NUTRITION DETOX PLAN

"We LOVE Risa's 14-Day Detox! So much so that we decided to extend it and go another round! We experienced decreased fatigue, increased energy and mental clarity, relief from joint stiffness and more restful sleep. We have experienced not just weight loss, but the cessation of food cravings, reduction of joint stiffness, clearer skin—and minds—and off the chart energy! I know we all want a quick fix, but those programs never stick long term. Do yourself a favor and let Risa teach you how to heal from within!" Not to mention weight loss. And the best part? Because this isn't a "3-shake-a-day" program, real food is incorporated, and we were NEVER hungry! It's a personalized, holistic, realistic, science-based, common sense approach to health, healing, and wellness through the foods we eat.

--Jon and Elizabeth G.

Ridding the body of toxins is not only possible but critical for optimal health. When a new client comes into my office, 99 percent of the time I recommend that they start with my Risa Groux Nutrition Detox while waiting for their tests results to come in. I do this for many different reasons. Not only is it a swift way to start seeing results including weight loss, increased energy, and many times, a disappearance of pain, headaches, and inflammation, but it provides the proper nutrition and boundaries to start the healing process. It takes 14-21 days to break a habit, and this is the perfect way to jump in. Most people on the detox will come into my office during their second week and ask if they can continue because they feel so good and want to keep feeling that way.

I encourage you to detox as your first step because by simply removing some inflammatory foods and consuming healthy ones, symptoms will often vanish. Remember, decreasing systemic inflammation and increasing good gut health is always my goal--as that is usually the root of optimal health.

The program I developed, the Risa Groux Nutrition (RGN) Detox, is a 14-day whole food program to purify the body. It's *not* a diet--it's a kick-start to a new eating lifestyle like the Paleo FoodFrame you'll read about in Chapter 4 which eliminates gluten, dairy, sugar, grains, and legumes while including quality foods that promote daily excretion of toxins to prevent a toxic build-up. It is not calorie-restrictive, so you eat when you're hungry and don't eat when you're not feeling hungry. It removes cravings for sugar and processed carbohydrates. Along with two delicious collagen shakes per day, the eating plan is filled with quality protein, good fats, and absorbable fiber. Detoxing does not equate with starvation! I want you to eat when you are hungry and not eat when you aren't!

The results you'll get with this Detox are weight loss, of course, but it is designed to be a wellness program to clean out your system, decrease systemic inflammation, and increase good gut health. As you know by now, weight loss is a side effect of wellness. Other quite common results are increased energy, regularity, and elimination of bloating, digestion issues, joint pain, headaches, migraines, brain fog, and improved skin and mood.

TOXIN PRIMER

The Environmental Protection Agency (EPA) defines a toxic chemical as "any substance which may be harmful to the environment or hazardous to your health if inhaled, ingested, or absorbed through the skin." You can get toxins into your body three ways: Through foods we eat and beverages we drink, chemicals we breathe in, and the products we put on our skin.

Foods We Eat	**Chemicals We Breathe**	**What Meets Our Skin**
Additives	Air fresheners	Deodorant
Alcohol	Bug spray/repellant	Hair dyes
Coffee	Cigarette smoke	Hair styling products
Food coloring	Chemicals on masks	Makeup/cosmetics
Fried foods	Dyes and coloring	Nail polish/remover
High fructose corn syrup	Fabric, especially upholstery, bed sheets and pillowcases, clothing, window coverings, shower curtains, car upholstery, etc.	Shampoo/conditioner
Medication/Pharmaceuticals		Shaving cream
MSG		Sunscreen
Non-organic foods	Fire retardants	
Processed foods	Formaldehyde, from carpets/furniture	
Preservatives	Household cleaning supplies	
	Paint	
	Perfume/fragrance	
	Pesticides/herbicides/fertilizers	

Toxin Facts

*There are currently 82,000 FDA-approved chemicals registered for use in the US. Over 3,000 of them are sanctioned for consumption in food and beverages. That is a ludicrously huge number of chemicals! No other country on the planet has approved this enormous amount of chemicals for their citizens to use. And as you already know, your gut is where 75-85 percent of your immune system is produced. Our gut houses many immune cells in what's known as gut-associated lymphoid tissue. In addition, epithelial cells that line the intestines form a barrier that blocks destructive pathogens from entering the rest of the body and wreak damage.

The FDA has a long history of approving chemicals without proof of product safety. They approve roughly 2,000 chemicals per year. Unfortunately, many of those chemicals are not tested for their long-term impact on health nor are they tested by a third party unassociated with the company. It's the companies themselves who test their products and restrict the reporting of negative responses in their filings with the FDA. These reports are taken at face value by the FDA who rarely test any of the products oftentimes because of a lack of personnel and funding.

- Many of these chemicals can disrupt your body systems: immune, nervous, endocrine, and reproductive.
- Pesticides have been linked to a wide range of human health hazards, ranging from short-term impacts such as headaches and nausea to chronic impacts like cancer, reproductive harm, and endocrine disruption. They can also present acute dangers, such as nerve, skin, and eye irritation and damage; headaches, dizziness, nausea, fatigue, and systemic poisoning, and even occasionally fatal.
- The average American woman comes in contact with over 200 toxins before leaving the bathroom each day.
- Americans apply an average of 126 toxins on their skin each day absorbing 80 percent of them.
- Baby umbilical cords were found to have approximately 287 toxins in a recent research study,[4] meaning that babies are born with a toxic load.
- The food additive business had an estimated $45 billion in sales in 2018—even though food additives and preservatives can cause leaky gut, food allergies, food intolerance, cancer, multiple sclerosis, attention deficit hyperactivity disorder (ADHD), brain damage, nausea, cardiac disease, and more.
- Some natural preservatives such as ascorbic acid (vitamin C), garlic, lemon, sea salt or Himalayan salt, vinegar, or vitamin C can be used without side effects or damage to the body.

Toxin Effects

---

[4] "Body Burden: The Pollution in Newborns." EWG, www.ewg.org/research/body-burden-pollution-newborns.

What happens when you consume, absorb, or ingest toxins? Your liver needs to convert them into enzymes so it can process the toxins through digestion and elimination. Unfortunately, your liver cannot effectively process every toxin—so the excess is stored in fat cells and tissues. Once these toxins accumulate, they can have a negative impact on the entire body in a variety of ways.

Common symptoms of chronic toxicity include:

- Bloating and gas
- Canker sores and rashes
- Diarrhea/ constipation and foul-smelling stools/ other gastrointestinal problems
- Difficulty concentrating
- Eczema, acne, and skin issues
- Fatigue
- Food cravings/weight gain
- Headaches/migraines
- Inability to lose weight
- Low libido
- Joint pain and muscle aches
- Puffy dark circles under the eyes
- Reduced mental clarity
- Sinus congestion and chronic sinus issues
- Sleep issues

How to Determine Your Toxic Load

Your toxic load is the amount of toxins your body needs to process. By answering the following questions, you may gain some insight as to your current toxic load.

- Do you or have you eaten processed foods?
- Do you consume genetically altered food?
- Do you eat non-organic fruits and vegetables?
- Do you eat meat and poultry that are not free-range?
- Do you or have you ever used artificial sweeteners?
- Do you regularly drink soda?
- Do the foods you eat contain additives, dyes, preservatives, or sweeteners?
- Do you eat fast foods and/or eat out regularly?
- Do you charbroil or grill foods?
- Do you drink coffee regularly?
- Do you drink alcohol?
- Do you drink tap water?

If most of your answers are *yes*, then it is likely that what you consume contributes significantly to your toxic load. Beyond that, many external toxins, such as perfumes, cleaners, and pollution, add to your load. Your health care professional can help you assess your levels.

THE BENEFITS OF A DETOX

"I heard of Risa from my sister-in-law in Newport Beach. She had never really dieted, was always a health-conscious eater, and decided to try the RGN Detox. She kept telling me how great she was feeling, sleeping, and that the weight was falling off. Her arthritis was better and overall, that's what got me. She told Risa about me and Risa agreed to help me long distance! Risa did an extensive review process and ordered labs that I had never done before. She shared with me so many things

I hadn't been told by doctors and she put me on a plan. I obviously had a bad gut, a lot of inflammation, and some autoimmune issues.

A little about me: I am 59 years old and have struggled with IBS my whole life. I had followed many weight-loss plans only to gain it back again. It was always about the scale and clothes size for me until Risa! The cleanse sounded so restrictive. I had done many diets before but never got health benefits and results like this. After only two months I believe my stomach is healed. I go to the bathroom every day and I never thought I would say this but that is more important than the numbers on the scale. Risa put me on the elimination diet and I now am educated on what my body doesn't tolerate therefore I don't want to eat those things anymore. Feeling good trumps the bad food and alcohol.

The whole plan is a combination of Risa's knowledge and how she uses the labs results, supplements, and diet to heal your body. I have only done diets before but never experienced results like this. The supplements are amazing. I will stay on those for life. The protein shakes are a great way to start the day and I previously was a huge egg eater at breakfast! This is something that for the first time in my life I can stick to and that helps me enjoy my life. All to say, I am beyond grateful to have met Risa. She is a wonderful cheerleader, you know she really cares, and she gets so much joy out of helping others."

--Andi P.

Detoxifying, also known as purification or cleansing, can help you remove toxins from your body and helps maintain a healthy weight. A detox program can have a significant, positive effect on the biochemistry of your body while allowing natural toxins and byproducts of daily metabolism to be eliminated. It offers your body additional support to expel toxins and minimize your weight, which is important to maintaining health and vitality.

As you just read, we are exposed to external toxins every day, including pollutants, pesticides, and chemicals. Internally our bodies produce waste byproducts as a result of normal metabolic function. Although your body is designed to rid itself of these toxins naturally, it can become overburdened. With constant exposure to chemicals, even if you decrease your toxic load, it is essential for your body to detoxify from the chemicals that are stored in your fat cells and fat tissues.

Riding your body of toxins is not only possible but critical for optimal health—especially because boosting your immunity through detoxing and decreasing inflammation can help protect you from contracting viruses.

How to Reduce Your Toxic Load

It's not difficult to reduce your toxic load once you know what to do and what to look for.

<u>Eat as Many Organic and Non-GMO Foods as Possible</u>

Organic foods are farmed foods that are grown with little to no use of pesticides, herbicides, fungicides, and/or insecticides in the process. Eating them is a healthier choice, but organic labeling laws are overly complex and can be misleading. Many small organic growers cannot afford to have their products labeled as such because of the prohibitive cost and the hoops they have to jump through to have their products labelled as organic. When you go to the farmer's market, ask your produce provider about the methods they use to grow their foods. It's worth doing your homework, because:

- Organic food decreases or eliminates our toxic load.
- Some studies show that organic foods have more beneficial nutrients, such antioxidants, than their conventionally grown counterparts.
- People with allergies to foods, chemicals, or preservatives often find their symptoms lessen or go away when they eat organic
- Organic food is usually fresher because it doesn't contain preservatives that make it last longer. It's often produced on smaller farms near your community.
- Organically raised animals are not given antibiotics, growth hormones, or fed animal byproducts. Overuse of antibiotics helps create antibiotic-resistant strains of bacteria, which can be dangerous for you should you get an infection or illness.
- Organic food is usually GMO-free. Genetically Modified Organisms (GMOs) are plants or animals whose DNA has deliberately been altered, usually to make it pesticide or disease resistant.
- Organic farming is better for the environment because it reduces pollution, conserves water, reduces soil erosion, increases soil fertility, and uses less energy.
- Organic crops must be kept separate from conventional products and grown in safe soil that hasn't received modifications of any kind. This means that farmers are not allowed to use synthetic pesticides, bioengineered genes (GMOs), petroleum-based fertilizers, and sewage sludge-based fertilizers.

SIDEBAR – Produce that Should Always Be Organic

According to the Environmental Working Group, a nonprofit organization that analyzes the results of government pesticide testing in the US, the following 14 fruits and vegetables have the highest pesticide levels on average. Try to buy these as organic produce whenever possible:

- Apples
- Sweet Bell Peppers
- Cucumbers
- Celery
- Potatoes
- Grapes
- Cherry Tomatoes
- Kale/Collard Greens
- Summer Squash
- Nectarines (imported)
- Peaches
- Spinach
- Berries
- Hot Peppers

These conventionally grown foods tend to have lower pesticide levels.

- Asparagus
- Avocado
- Mushrooms
- Cabbage
- Sweet Corn
- Eggplant
- Kiwi
- Mango
- Onion
- Papaya
- Pineapple
- Sweet Peas (frozen)
- Sweet Potatoes
- Grapefruit
- Cantaloupe

Eat Grass-Fed and Grass-Finished Meat

Cattle are meant to eat grass in fields and pastures, when they do, they tend to be healthier and leaner, and grass-fed beef has been shown to have higher levels of healthy omega-3 fatty acids. Just be aware that meat labeled as grass-fed but *not* certified organic may have been raised on pasture exposed to or treated with pesticides or fertilizers.

In addition, despite all the label regulations we have in place, cattle farmers were able to find loopholes. They realized that even though federal regulations state that you should feed a cow grass for its lifetime, it is legal to feed it grain for the last thirty days of its life for the sole purpose of fattening it up before slaughter. This improves profit margins for the farmers and allows them to still qualify as grass-fed. These animals are likely fed massive quantities of corn and soy (most commonly GMO) to make them a lot bigger.

To avoid this loophole, look for meat that is labeled grass-fed *and* grass-finished, which can be found in specialty stores like Whole Foods and selected butchers.

Eat Free-Range and Pastured Poultry

Free-range gives consumers the impression that these chickens or turkeys were allowed to spend their lives free roaming in large fields, but all it means is that the animals weren't confined to a cage and had access to the outdoors for brief periods of time. And the terms free-range or free-roaming also don't apply to egg-laying hens. So, if you can find eggs at a local farmers' market, you can ask the farmers directly about their practices.

Eat Wild-Caught Fish

In recent years, there has been a huge decline in many species of fish due to unsustainable fishing and farming practices. Unfortunately, there are several health reasons not to eat farmed fish:

- Farmed fish are higher in Omega6 fatty acids which promote inflammation. Wild fish are higher in Omega3 fatty acids which *reduces* inflammation.
- Due to crowded conditions, farmed fish are fed antibiotics to prevent disease from killing the fish.
- Cancer causing chemicals such as PCBs are found in farmed salmon in significantly higher levels than wild salmon--reported to be up to 816 times higher.

It's always better to eat wild-caught fish that have been sustainably caught—it will say so on the packaging.

In addition, you need to be aware that common toxins such as mercury are often found in fish. That's because dangerous quantities of mercury are emitted into the air and dumped into waterways thanks to widespread industrial waste. When it rains, the toxins that are in the air fall into our lakes and oceans where it further contaminates fish and shellfish. Mercury is a poison that interferes with the brain and nervous system, and it can cause serious health problems. The bigger the fish, like shark or tuna, the higher the mercury levels. Nursing mothers, pregnant women, and young children are at higher risk, and should avoid all large fish (shark, swordfish, king mackerel, tilefish, and ahi tuna).

Drink Clean Spring Water or Reverse Osmosis Water

And drink a lot of it every day!

When I moved into our family home, I did my research and purchased the most expensive and highly recommended water filtration system to be installed under my kitchen sink. It was attached to a separate faucet for cooking with cold and instant hot water that was installed just for my top-of-the-line water filtration system. It tasted pretty clean, but I wanted to make sure, so I purchased a water meter to calculate the contaminants in my water. I was so eager to see the results when the meter arrived, as it measured a variety of contaminants with a maximum number of 500. Initially I tested the unfiltered tap water which came in at 489. My excitement was immediately tampered when I discovered that my elite filtration system showed up for 478 contaminants! I retested a few times on separate days just to make sure but got the same results. I promptly purchased a reverse osmosis machine and had it installed. The new reading for my filtered water was now 11, and I was overjoyed! These little changes really add up, so I encourage you to drink clean water.

Use Beauty Products with as Few Chemicals as Possible

There are so many choices available for skincare, hair care, and makeup that it's very difficult to know what's best for your body. Look for products without parabens, sulfurs, or aluminums. The Environmental Working Group has an immensely helpful "Skin-Deep Guide to Cosmetics" on their website (https://www.ewg.org/skindeep/) so you can make informed choices.

Results of Your Detox

By participating in a cleansing program, you're likely to notice the following:

- Better focus and elimination of brain fog
- Better mood
- Clearer skin
- Decrease or elimination of headaches
- Elimination of joint pain
- Elimination of sugar and carb cravings
- Increased energy
- Bowel regularity
- Weight loss

Remember: Mainstream medicine does not really consider toxins or toxic load as it relates to health nor do most mainstream practitioners know much about them as they were never taught this topic in medical school. After seeing countless people regain their health and vitality in my office, day after day, I am fully confident in the enormous contribution that toxins play in illness—as well as the benefits of detoxifying the proper way.

Juice "Cleanses" Are *Not* Detoxes!

Go to any health-food store and you will see shelves laden with different cleanses, whether they're from juice, colonic, lemon and cayenne, or supplements in a bottle. Most juices contain some beneficial nutrients—but only if they are organic and only if they are consumed within hours of extraction. Most of them, however, are filled with sugar from fruits so they taste good—and you order more!

These cleanses all have the same detox goal but are not necessarily effective or right for everyone. I have probably tried them all. I've forced down sludge-like liquids and supplements paired with daily colonics, and experimented with store-bought cleanses, which were equally ineffective. So, let me tell you why these cleanses are only good for lightening your wallet!

- I prefer to call raw juice cleanses "juice fasts" as they contain absolutely no fiber, the indigestible part of plant foods, which is absolutely essential to clean anything out of your digestive system--consequently defeating the purpose of a cleanse! Fiber also reduces cholesterol and regulates sugar intake. Juice cleanses will give your digestive tract a break for a day--which is helpful from time to time--but their lack of fibers means they won't be getting rid of toxins.
- What you'll ingest are the micronutrients (vitamins and minerals) from the fruit or veggies, but without the mitigating effect of fiber, the concentrated sugar will spike your blood sugar levels. This can be a real problem if you are hypoglycemic or have diabetes.
- Most juices are extracted 1-4 days prior to you buying them. The efficacy of the enzymes minimizes within a few hours of extraction while the potential for bacterial growth of organisms increases, which leaves you with little more than expensive sugar water in a fancy bottle.
- Many juice cleanses are not organic, so instead of extracting toxins out of the body, there provide a steady flow of toxins entering the body.
- The "Master Cleanse" is one of those cleanses that just will not disappear. During the 7-10 days of misery when you're on it, all you can consume is water with lemon juice, maple syrup, and cayenne pepper. When I tried it years ago, it literally made me pass out. Trust me—it's not effective. I believe you need calories to function, and this "cleanse" puts your body in starvation mode, so you'll gain even more weight when you go off it as your metabolism has slowed down. There is a big difference between fasting and starving, and I don't believe a long-term fast is right for most.

THE RGN DETOX IS BEST

Because so many of the cleanses and detoxes available to the public are ineffective, I decided to create my own. Since I do so much whole-food detoxing with my clients and see the incredible results--not just weight loss but regained health and vitality--I knew that coming up with the right elements was critical, especially for non-GMO, gluten, dairy, and soy-free ingredients. I launched the RGN Detox and the results started pouring in immediately. People love it! They really enjoy the structure of the food plan, especially the shakes and how satisfying they are, and what it includes and eliminates. Clients also rave about the convenience of the collagen protein and supplement packets which are individually packaged as an easy grab-and-go, simplifying dining out and traveling. Most importantly, they love how they feel when taking them. Weight loss is usually the common initial motivator, but in addition to that, people are ecstatic about the health benefits they start seeing typically during week two. Ninety percent of the people I work with ask to extend the detox to 28 days because they feel so good. Many people, in fact, detox several times throughout the year.

Now more than ever we need our immune system working for us, not against us. If we have a healthy balanced microbiome, it is much more difficult to host a virus, so people have been detoxing in droves. If there was ever a time to discuss genuine health, a global pandemic is it. Nothing will be more effective than maintaining a healthy body through natural foods, by decreasing your toxic load, and living a lifestyle to balance it all. I know I keep mentioning it, but I really want you to understand that most of our immune system is produced in our gut, so it's critical to create and maintain a healthy gut or microbiome. We do this by taking out the trash and replenishing the body with nourishing and healing foods.

Remember, we know that genetics play a part in disease but there are multiple factors in our control such as toxic load, nutrition, exercise, and lifestyle issues such as stress, sleep, and happiness. Changes in your lifestyle can be more effective than medication. I see it all the time.

The RGN Detox is designed to decrease systemic inflammation, increase good gut health, and restore vital nutrients so that all your organs can work optimally. The detox cleanses the body by removing many potential allergenic foods so you can get the best results and focus on purifying your body. Eating low toxic and anti-inflammatory food and taking the right kind of targeted supplements to aid in opening detoxifying pathways is the best way to go.

This short detox is the reset you need to remove carbs and sugars from your diet, cleaning your body, and losing weight. Practically everyone could benefit from removing toxins in their bodies, that is why I encourage you to do the detox as your first step. The new eating lifestyle on the detox will be a springboard for most FoodFrames in this book, so it's an easy place to start. In addition, you will feel better right away and start seeing results. It's an amazing body wake-up for anyone over the age of sixteen. It can be done up to four times annually.

The goal is healthy, not hungry--starvation has nothing to do with detoxifying! The RGN Detox is not calorie-restrictive, so I recommend eating if you're hungry and not eating when you're not... it is that simple. Most people find they're not very hungry while on the detox as they are getting all the required servings of protein, fat, and fiber. When you fill your gas tank to full, it doesn't require any more gas. Just like a car, your body won't ask for more nutrients when it gets enough of what it needs.

WHAT YOU GET WITH THE RGN DETOX

Once you receive the kit, you will find:

The Basics

- Two collagen shakes per day
- 28 single-serve collagen protein packets (for your collagen shakes)
- 28 supplement packets containing three RGN Detox capsules and one RGN Antiox capsule. These supplements contain amino acids and antioxidants to support Phase I and II for proper liver detoxification
- Detox booklet with guidelines, list of foods to include, list of foods to eliminate, delicious and easy recipes, and suggestions for meals, shakes, and snacks
- BPA-free shaker cup to conveniently take your shakes on the go with you

All products included are gluten, dairy, and soy-free and non-GMO.

The RGN Collagen Protein Powder

Collagen is the most abundant protein we have, accounting for 30 percent of the protein in our bodies and 70 percent of the protein in our skin. Comprised of many amino acids--the critical ones being proline, glycine, arginine, and glutamine--collagen is responsible for our skin's elasticity, the binding of our bones and muscles, and protection of our organs. It's also critical for the structure of joints and tendons as a component of connective tissues. But as we age, collagen production slows down significantly, contributing to wrinkles, aging skin, joint pain, diminished eye health, thinning hair, weak nails, digestive issues, and cellulite.

The RGN Collagen Protein benefits are:

- Building of muscle, cartilage, and ligaments
- Decreased joint pain
- Hair and nail growth
- Improved wound healing
- Increased gut health, improved digestion
- Increased immunity
- Reduced signs of skin aging, improved elasticity

Each serving contains:

- 18 grams of protein per serving to help maintain muscle during the detoxification program, and to fuel the liver enzyme systems that drive the detoxification process, in a highly concentrated and pure broth protein isolate

- Delicious berry-vanilla flavor with a wonderful, smooth texture; mixes easily in any liquid base of coconut milk, unsweetened almond milk, or water
- Free of dairy, gluten, soy, and lactose; sweetened with the herb stevia

The RGN Detox Capsules

- Supports effective phases I and II liver detoxification, which is essential to prevent the production of intermediate metabolites that could cause symptoms or sensitivity reactions during a detoxification program
  Note: Phase 1 detoxification occurs when oxidation take place, meaning the body will break down unhealthy toxins into less harmful metabolites. Antioxidants are critical during this process.
- Nutritional support for phase II detoxification helps conjugate (or extract) toxins from fat cells and prepare them for safe elimination from the body
  Note: Phase 2 detoxification is about extraction which uses several pathways to excrete the phase 1 metabolites out of the body. Amino acids are essential during this process.

The RGN Antiox Capsules

- Synergistically combines an extensive array of nutrients that combat free radicals and help support the detoxification of chemicals and heavy metals
- Contains multiple nutrients known to raise glutathione levels, making it helpful for supporting phase II liver detoxification. Glutathione is the master antioxidant we produce naturally; it's also a common supplement that I recommend for those with autoimmune conditions or inflammation of any kind. I take it daily and you might want to consider it as a possible protective aid against COVID-19 or any other internal or external attacks.

WHO SHOULD AVOID THIS DETOX

The RGN Detox is great for virtually anyone except pregnant or nursing women as we don't want the baby to get any toxins being purged out of the mother's body either the bloodstream in pregnancy or through breast milk. In addition, those who are very ill may not be strong enough to detox and I don't want to cause more harm. I do work with plenty of very ill people, but we go slowly on the detox, with one shake and one packet of supplements per day. The detox is quite effective most of the time but listen to your body as it will usually let you know how it's feeling.

If you have a lot of health issues or complications, I recommend working with a functional healthcare provider or physician who can guide and support you before starting any detox program. I would also recommend that seniors, those who are exposed to higher levels of chemicals at work, or individuals who eat a highly processed diet, slowly ease into it. Start with one shake and one packet of supplements per day instead of two. Once you feel ready, increase the shakes and supplement packets to twice daily.

It is not unusual to feel a slight bit sluggish the first few days as your body is hard at work riding itself of toxins. Many people don't feel any different at all, but either way you should start seeing an increase in energy starting at day five. If you do feel "off" for a few days, that usually means you have a lot to detox, but each time you detox thereafter, it gets easier. Many people experience an increase in the frequency of bowel movement, typically one or two more times throughout the day than usual; others see an increase in volume; and some see no change at all. This is all normal. You should not experience any urgency to go or any diarrhea.

Be patient and kind with yourself! You are giving your body the best gift, that of detoxing and rebooting. Get good quality sleep and rest if needed, but you should have enough energy to continue your exercise routine. The benefits *will* follow.

SIDEBAR – Freddie's Story

Out of the blue one fine day in 2018, I received a call from the world-famous PGA golfer Fred Couples and his physician who'd been referred to me by his physical therapist. They told me that Freddie needed to lose 20 pounds before the Masters in a few short months and asked if I could help him. Of course, I instantly agreed!

When Freddie came into my office and sat down, he winced. Over the years, he'd often talked about his intractable back pain, so when I asked him about it, he told me it would get slightly better from time to time, but that it was a chronic nuisance and he'd be thrilled to cross it off his list. He added that he also had smell sensitivity and regular headaches. He had tried seemingly every treatment and seen doctors from around the globe, and had been told he didn't need surgery, but no one had been able to help him. Playing golf every day was his job, but it also compounded the pain. On a scale of 1-10, with 10 being off-the-chart excruciating, Freddie told me that he was never under a seven or eight. Every day. That simply had to stop.

I immediately ordered extensive blood and stool tests to determine if Freddie's debilitating pain was from inflammation or something else. I had my suspicions that at least some of it could have been caused by exposure to outdoor herbicides and pesticides used to treat the golf course greens he walked on throughout his career—chemicals known to have serious health repercussions. That was a fairly simple deduction to make as none of the countless medical professionals he'd consulted over the years had diagnosed his pain as structural—so he'd never had surgery. I also put him on the RGN Detox, and when he returned the following week for his first check-in appointment, he happily told me that yes, he'd already lost four pounds, and his pain was down to a four. At that point, he was sure the Detox had nothing to do with his reduced pain, so I encouraged him to keep going. At his second appointment a week later, he told me his pain was at a one.

"How did you do that?" he asked. "I haven't felt like this in *years*!"

"Well, all those tests I ordered while you were detoxing confirmed my suspicions that you had systemic inflammation," I told him. "That's why I gave you large doses of natural anti-inflammatory supplements, mainly turmeric, along with the Paleo FoodFrame and the daily collagen shakes."

The Detox can be enjoyed for up to 28 days, and Fred begged me to allow him to stay on it for another two weeks. I agreed, and he continued to be 100% compliant. He also became more conscious of his food choices while on the road and at home—and he lost those 20 pounds. Even though he is on the road a tremendous amount of time, he made it work. His smell sensitivity and headaches disappeared. The sports announcers enjoyed a good chat with him about it during the Masters broadcast, especially as his golf scores improved as well. That may have been a coincidence, but I tend to think not.

And now, whenever I see Fred, I ask him what his number is.

He smiles and says, "It's a zero--unless I pick up a golf club, and then it's a one!"

DETOX FOODS TO ENJOY

Poultry

Includes broth and collagen

NOTE: Collagen can be found in bone broth that has been cooked for 24-48 hours. Bone broth is wonderful to cook with, and it's a perfect snack to sip for its continued benefits throughout the day.

Chicken, duck, goose, grouse, guinea hen, ostrich, pheasant, quail, turkey

Fish

Includes broth and collagen

Anchovy, arctic char, bass, bonito, carp, catfish, cod, eel, gar, haddock, hake, halibut, herring, mackerel, mahi-mahi, marlin, monkfish, perch, pollock, salmon, sardine, snapper, sole, swordfish, tilapia, trout, tuna, ahi, yellowfin, turbot, walleye

Shellfish

Includes broth and collagen

Clams, crab, crawfish, lobster, mussels, octopus, oysters, scallops, shrimp, squid

Eggs

Chicken, duck, goose, quail, including fish eggs/caviar

Leafy Vegetables

Unlimited

Arugula, beet greens, Bok choy, broccoli rabe, Brussels sprouts, cabbage, carrot tops, celery, chicory, collard greens, cress, dandelion greens, endive, all varieties of kale, all varieties of lettuce, mustard greens, Napa cabbage, purslane, radicchio, sorrel, spinach, Swiss chard, turnip greens, watercress

Non-starchy Vegetables

Unlimited

Artichoke, asparagus, broccoli, cauliflower, celery, fennel, kohlrabi, rhubarb, squash blossoms, water chestnuts

Allium-family Vegetables

Chive, garlic, leek, onion, scallion, shallot, wild leek

Roots, Tubers, and Bulb Vegetables

In moderation

Arrowroot, bamboo shoot, beet, burdock, cassava, rutabaga, sweet potato (maximum half daily), taro, turnip, wasabi, yam (maximum half daily), carrot, celeriac, daikon, ginger, horseradish, lotus root, jicama, parsnip, radish, yam noodles

Nightshades or Spices Derived from Nightshades

Omit if Autoimmune (see Chapter 5)

Ashwagandha, capsicums/bell and sweet peppers, chili pepper flakes, chili powder, paprika, cayenne pepper, jalapeno, chipotle, and red pepper, hot peppers, pepinos, and pimentos; cape gooseberries, eggplant, goji berries (wolfberries), potatoes (sweet potatoes and yams are not nightshades and are okay), sweet plantains, tomatoes (all varieties)

Sea Vegetables

Arame, dulse, hijiki, kombu, nori, wakame

Vegetable-like Fruits

Avocado, bitter melon, chayote, cucumber, okra, olives, plantain (in moderation), pumpkin, squash, winter melon, zucchini

Berries

0-1 serving daily if not pre-diabetic/diabetic

Blackberry, blueberry, cranberry, raspberry, strawberry

Citrus-family Fruits

Lemon, lime

Other Fruits

In moderation

Banana (¼-⅓ maximum), coconut (all varieties, unsweetened), ½ apple (omit if SIBO is present)

Edible Fungi/Mushrooms

Chanterelle, cremini, morel, oyster, porcini, portobello, shiitake, truffle

Animal Fats

Bacon fat, butter, ghee, lard, pan drippings, poultry fat, chicken, or goose fat, strutto (clarified pork fat), tallow (from beef, lamb, or mutton)

Plant Fats

Avocado oil (cold-pressed), coconut oil, extra virgin olive oil (cold-pressed), flaxseed oil, sesame oil, walnut oil

Nuts/Nut Butters and Nut Oils

Almonds, Brazil nuts, chestnuts, hazelnuts, macadamia, pistachios, pecans, pine nuts, walnuts

Seeds and Seed Oils

Chia, flax, hemp, poppy, pumpkin, sesame, sunflower

Probiotic Foods

Fermented poultry or fish, kimchi, kombucha, lacto-fermented vegetables, sauerkraut

Herbs and Spices

*Watch for added ingredients

Allspice, anise, annatto, basil leaf, bay leaf, black caraway, cardamom, celery seed, chamomile, Chinese five-spice powder, chervil, chives, cilantro, coriander, cinnamon, cloves, cumin, curry powder, dill, fennel seed, fennel leaf, fenugreek, garlic, ginger, garam masala, juniper, kaffir lime leaf, lavender, lemongrass, mace, marjoram leaf, mustard, nutmeg, onion powder, oregano leaf, parsley, pepper, peppermint, poppy, rosemary, saffron, sage, savory leaf, sea or Himalayan salt, spearmint, tarragon, thyme, truffles, turmeric, vanilla

Flavorings

*Watch for added ingredients and sugar

Anchovies or anchovy paste, apple cider vinegar, balsamic vinegar, capers, carob powder, coconut aminos (a soy sauce substitute), coconut concentrate, red wine vinegar, truffle oil (made with olive oil), white wine vinegar

Sweeteners

*In moderation

Allulose, erythritol, mannitol, monk fruit (Luo Han Guo), raw honey (maximum 1 tablespoon), sorbitol, stevia, xylitol

Beverages

Water: club, mineral, reverse osmosis, seltzer, soda, sparkling, (without sweeteners or additives), spring, almond milk (unsweetened), coconut water (in moderation), coconut milk (unsweetened), hemp milk (unsweetened), herbal teas

Foods and Beverages Included in Moderation

Caffeinated teas (if reducing coffee intake), freshly squeezed green juices (without fruit), polyunsaturated fat-rich foods (poultry and industrially raised fatty meat)

DETOX FOODS TO AVOID

Meat

Excludes broth or collagen

Cattle (beef, veal), deer (venison), goat, hare, pig (pork), rabbit, sheep (lamb, mutton), wild game (buffalo/bison, boar, elk)

Dairy

Buttermilk, cheese (all types), cream (all varieties), curds, dairy-protein isolates, ice cream, kefir, milk, whey in any form, yogurt (all types, including Greek, unless homemade coconut or Nut-based and unsweetened)

Grains and Grain-Like Foods

Amaranth, barley, buckwheat, bulgur, corn, farro, millet, oats/oatmeal, quinoa, rice, wild rice, rye, sorghum, spelt, teff, wheat (all varieties, including einkorn and semolina)

Legumes

Adzuki beans, black beans, black-eyed peas, butter beans, calico beans, cannellini beans, chickpeas (garbanzo beans), fava beans (broad beans), great northern beans, green beans, Italian beans, kidney beans, lentils, lima beans, mung beans, navy beans, peanuts, peas, pinto beans, soybeans (including edamame, tofu, tempeh, soy sauce, other soy products, and soy isolates, such as soy lecithin), split peas

Berries

Acai, currant, elderberry, gooseberry, grapes (all varieties), lingonberry, mulberry

Rosaceae-family Fruits

Apricot, cherry, nectarine, peach, pear, plum, quince, rosehip

Melons

Cantaloupe, honeydew, horned melon, melon pear, Persian melon, watermelon, winter melon

Citrus-family Fruits

Clementine, grapefruit, kumquat, orange, pomelo, tangelo, tangerine, yuzu

Tropical Fruits

Fresh and dried

Acerola, chayote, cherimoya, date, dragon fruit, durian, fig, guava, jackfruit, kiwi, loquat, lychee, mango, mangosteen, papaya, passion fruit, pawpaw, persimmon, pineapple, pomegranate, raisins, star fruit, tamarind

Nuts/Nut Butters and Nut Oils

Cashews, peanuts

Probiotic Foods

Fermented meat, kombucha, kvass, lacto-fermented fruits, non-dairy and dairy kefir

Plant Fats

Palm oil, palm shortening

Processed Vegetable Oils

Canola oil (rapeseed oil), corn oil, cottonseed oil, grapeseed oil, palm kernel oil, peanut oil, safflower oil, soybean oil, sunflower oil

Flavorings

Chutneys, jam, jellies

Processed Food Chemicals and Ingredients

Acrylamides, any ingredient with an unrecognizable chemical name, artificial and natural flavors, artificial food color, autolyzed protein, brominated vegetable oil, emulsifiers (carrageenan, cellulose gum, guar gum, lecithin), hydrolyzed vegetable protein, monosodium glutamate, nitrates or nitrites (naturally occurring are okay), olestra, phosphoric acid, propylene glycol, textured vegetable protein (TVP), trans fats (partially hydrogenated vegetable oil, hydrogenated oil), yeast extract

Sugars

Agave, agave nectar, barley malt, barley malt syrup, beet sugar, brown rice syrup, brown sugar, cane crystals, cane juice, cane sugar, raw cane sugar, evaporated cane juice, dehydrated cane juice, caramel, coconut sugar, coconut syrup, corn sweetener, corn syrup, corn syrup solids, crystalline fructose, date sugar, demerara sugar, dextrin, dextrose, fructose, high-fructose corn syrup, fruit juice, fruit juice concentrate, glucose, glucose solids, golden syrup, invert sugar, jaggery, lactose, lucuma, malt syrup, maltodextrin, maltose, maple sugar, maple syrup, molasses, muscovado sugar, palm sugar, raw sugar, refined sugar, rice bran syrup, rice syrup, saccharose, sorghum syrup, sucanat, sucrose, syrup, treacle, turbinado sugar, yacon syrup

Artificial Sweeteners

Acesulfame potassium, aspartame (Sweet 'n Low, Equal), neotame, saccharin, sucralose (Splenda)

Alcohol

All beer, liquor, wine, or any other form of alcoholic beverages are not permitted while detoxing

Beverages

Coffee (decaf and caffeinated), coconut water, cow milk, dairy-based kefir, energy drinks, electrolyte drinks, fruit juices, oat milk, rice milk, sodas (diet and regular), soymilk, sports drinks, oat milk, yerba mate; any drinks containing artificial coloring, flavors, sweeteners, or preservatives

LIFE AFTER THE DETOX

Once you've completed the Risa Groux Nutrition Detox, I recommend staying on the collagen protein shakes for breakfast each morning or perhaps an optional second one later in the day. The collagen protein that's suggested after detoxing is straight collagen as opposed to the collagen protein packets with additional nutrients to aid in the detoxifying process. Many people I work with love the routine of two shakes a day and not having to think about or plan too much around their food. The collagen shake for breakfast will not only start your day with a nutrient-dense meal that is satiating but will continue to give you the benefits of weight loss and optimal health.

Chocolate and vanilla flavors along with shake recipes are available at www.RisaGrouxNutrition.com. You can also have eggs for breakfast once or twice a week. or other breakfast items if desired. But the collagen shake is delicious, filling, easy, and provides all the powerhouse macro and micronutrients you need to start your day.

As for other food moving forward, I recommend eating the exact same foods that served you so well on the detox and making sure you have protein, fat, and fiber at every meal. You can now start adding back some other foods:

- Beef, lamb, pork (in moderation), or any other meats that were not permitted on the detox. The RGN Detox is intended to ease digestion, so these meats were removed because they can be difficult to digest. If you find them difficult to digest, I recommend taking one Enzyme Max with each meal. It is a combination of digestive enzymes to help break down proteins, carbs, and fat.
- Natural sugars like honey, coconut sugar and maple syrup are also allowed back in moderation. Remember even though they are natural, they are still sugars and will spike blood sugar levels--so go easy!
- Flours such as coconut, almond, hazelnut, cassava, or other Paleo-permitted flours. These are clean baking flours which you are perfectly welcome to enjoy but note they do contain carbohydrates. Use in moderation if you are aiming for weight loss.
- Coffee is usually a tough one. If you must bring your coffee back in, I recommend that you drink organic coffee, as conventional beans are heavily sprayed with pesticides. If you are among the millions who have a love affair with your coffee all day, aim for one cup in the morning.
There is very controversial research regarding coffee and its health benefits as well as its detriments, but my research and personal experience with clients shows that if you don't have an adrenal or autoimmune issue, you are good with having a cup of organic coffee every day. After all, it's often what people put into their coffee that's the culprit. If you need cream

and sugar, please use real food! Coconut cream or milk, unsweetened almond milk, and stevia, monk fruit, or allulose. If you like chocolate, use raw cacao. No chemical-laden creamers, artificial sweeteners, sugar, or sugary syrups, and certainly no whipped cream and sprinkles!

- Alcohol can often be particularly challenging to give up, even if only for fourteen days. Alcohol does not help your liver; in fact, it promotes a fatty liver. In addition, beer contains gluten which is inflammatory and damages the villi in the intestinal lining, which can lead to leaky gut. No matter what kind of alcohol you drink, it turns into sugar in your body, which will hinder weight loss and increase inflammation. In other words, alcohol can pack on the pounds. One glass of wine can be detected on the scale for up to four days after consumption—not necessarily because you have gained weight, but rather because of the sugars and gut inflammation that cause gas and bloating usually show up. I see this with my clients all the time. In addition to weight gain, many wines have added sulfites, yeast, additives, preservatives, dyes, and even sugars to enhance flavor and shelf life.

If you really need to have a glass of wine, I recommend an organic, low sugar, and clean version. There are new brands of wine, such as Dry Farms or Fit Vine, that are a much better choice. Read the label and know what's going inside your body. Or, if you would rather enjoy a cocktail, I would recommend going with the lowest sugar and cleanest form of liquor as possible--which puts most tequila, vodka, or gin at the top of that list. Enjoy your drink in moderation with some sparkling water, lemon, or lime. If you like it sweet, add stevia, monk fruit, or allulose.

Now that you have been putting leather, rubber and canvas in your sneaker factory and your body is functioning more optimally, think about what you really want. If you really want alcohol, then have it and enjoy it--but don't have it just because it's there or you feel social pressure. I'm all about balance, and life is no fun without things we enjoy, so just like you budget your money and your time, budget your food and your alcohol. Avoiding all alcohol after your detox for as long as you can manage is the perfect opportunity to give your liver a big hug. Trust me, alcohol will always be there!

RGN DETOX RECIPES

Detox Berry Shake

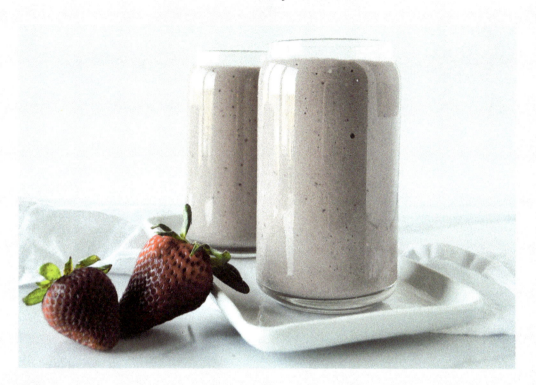

Ingredients:

1 cup coconut milk
1 packet of RGN Detox Collagen Protein
1-2 handfuls organic greens
½ cup organic strawberries (fresh or frozen) or ¼ avocado
1 handful ice, if not using frozen berries

Instructions:

Place all ingredients in a blender and blend until smooth.

Serves 1

Detox Greenie Shake

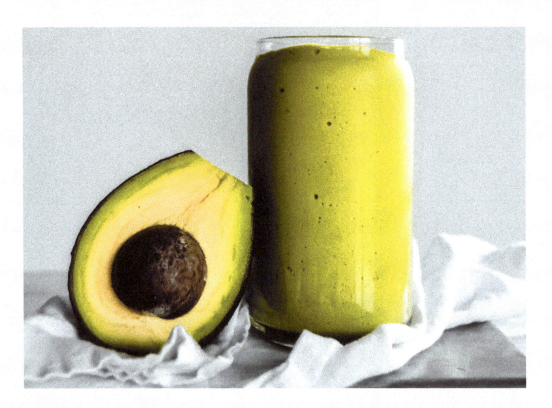

🧪 Ingredients:

1 cup almond milk
1 Packet of RGN Detox Collagen Protein
1 handful of spinach
½ fresh avocado
1 teaspoon chia seeds
1 cup ice

🧪 Instructions:

Place all ingredients in a blender and blend until smooth.

Serves 1

Warm Brussels Sprout Caesar Salad

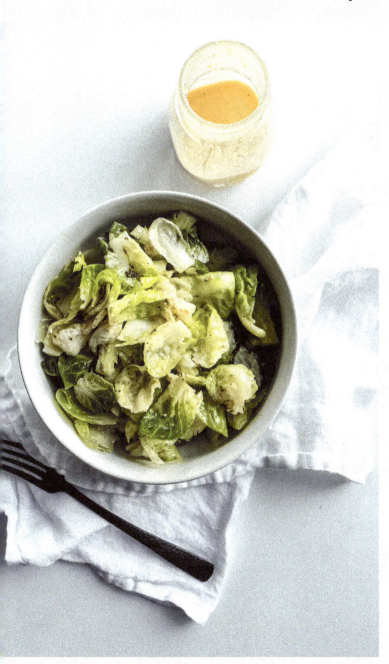

🍴 Ingredients:

1 pound of Brussels sprouts
2 teaspoons coconut or avocado oil
freshly ground black pepper

Caesar Dressing:
¼ cup extra-virgin olive oil
½ teaspoon lemon zest
2 tablespoons fresh lemon juice
1 large garlic clove
1 heaping teaspoon Dijon mustard
1 teaspoon coconut aminos
Sea salt and pepper to taste

🍴 Instructions:

1. Cut the Brussels sprouts in half from the top to the stem end, then thinly slice them crosswise.
2. In a large skillet, heat the oil over medium high heat, add the sliced Brussels sprouts and sauté until heated through and just beginning to wilt. They will have a nice green color. (Approximately 3-5 minutes).
3. In a blender or food processor, combine the oil, lemon zest and juice, garlic, mustard, and coconut aminos. Blend until smooth. Season with salt and pepper to taste.
4. Toss some of the dressing with the Brussels sprouts and serve.

Dressing can be made four days ahead.

Serves 4

Ahi Poke

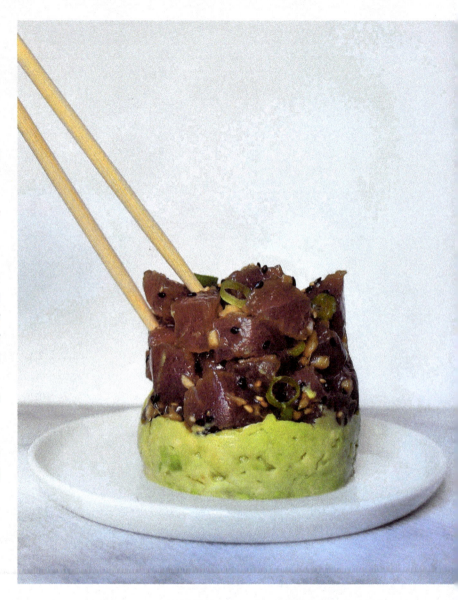

Ingredients:

1 lb. fresh wild ahi tuna steak, cubed
¼ cup scallions, chopped
1 teaspoon fresh ginger, minced
1 ½ tablespoons coconut aminos
1 tablespoon toasted sesame oil
1 teaspoon black and/or white toasted sesame seeds

Optional: 2 teaspoons tobiko or masago

Instructions:

1. Combine all ingredients in a medium sized bowl and gently mix. Cover and refrigerate for a couple of hours to meld the flavors together.
2. Garnish with additional sesame seeds, green onions, and serve.

Serve as an appetizer with cucumber slices or chips or on a bed of mashed avocado.

Serves 4

Jicama Fries

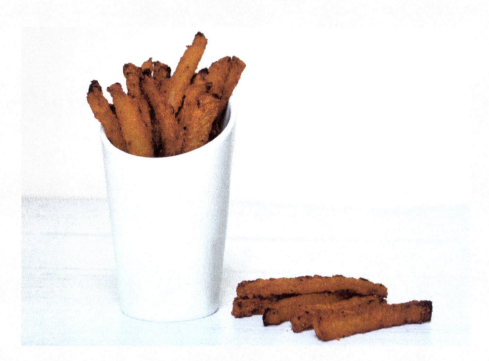

Ingredients:

1 jicama (approximately 1 pound), peeled and cut into ¼ inch thick fries

1 tablespoon olive oil

½ teaspoon sea salt

½ teaspoon smoked paprika

¼ teaspoon freshly ground black pepper

Instructions:

1. Place jicama fries in a large pot filled with two to three inches of water and heat on medium high for about 20-25 minutes.
2. Preheat oven to 400 degrees. Place a cooling rack on a cookie sheet.
3. In a large bowl, toss the jicama fries with the olive oil and the spices until fully covered. Arrange on the cooling rack and bake for 45 minutes until browned, turning halfway through.
4. To make it crispier, broil for the remaining 5 minutes.

Serve immediately.

Serves 4-8

Roasted Tomato Basil Soup

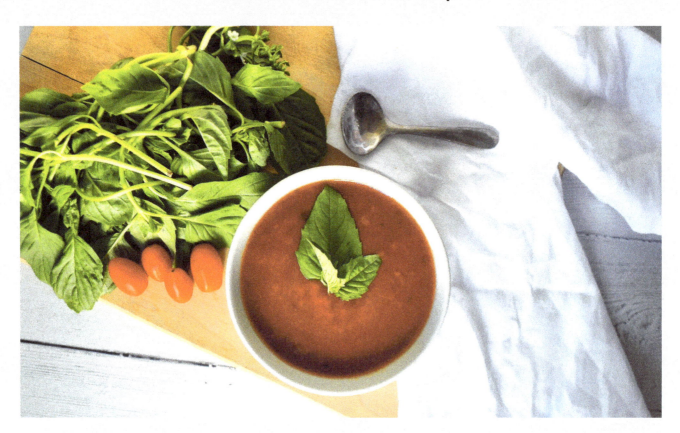

🍴 Ingredients:

3 pounds ripe plum tomatoes cut in half
¼ cup plus 2 tablespoons of olive oil
2 cups chopped yellow onions (about 2 small onions or 1 large)
6 garlic cloves, minced

28-ounce jar or can of plum tomatoes with liquid
4 cups fresh basil leaves, packed
1 teaspoon fresh (or dried) thyme leaves
1 quart of chicken or vegetable broth
Sea salt and pepper to taste

Optional: ¼ teaspoon crushed red pepper flakes

Instructions:

Preheat oven to 400 degrees.

1. Toss the fresh tomatoes with ¼ cup olive oil. Spread the tomatoes in a single layer on a baking sheet and roast for 45 minutes.
2. In an 8-quart stockpot over medium heat, sauté the onions, garlic, and red pepper flakes for 10 minutes until the onions start to brown.
3. Add jarred tomatoes, basil, thyme, and chicken (or vegetable) broth.
4. Add the oven-roasted tomatoes including the liquid on the baking sheet. Bring to a boil and simmer uncovered for 40 minutes.
5. Using a hand blender to blend thoroughly. Add sea salt and pepper to taste.

Garnish with a basil leaf or a sprinkle of chopped basil.

Serves 4-6

Grilled Herb Chicken

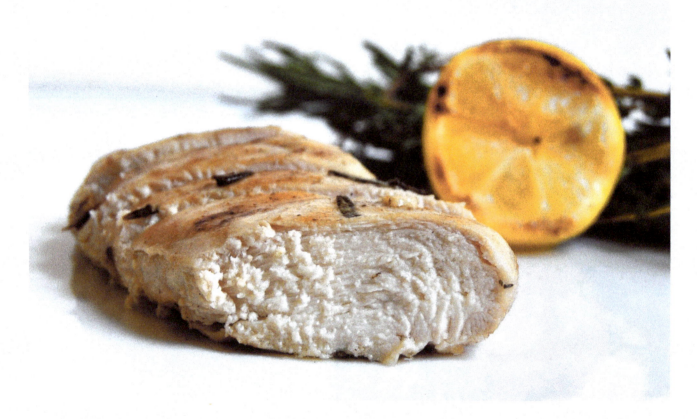

🍴 Ingredients:

3 tablespoons fresh lemon juice
2 tablespoons minced garlic
1 tablespoon chopped fresh rosemary
1 tablespoon chopped fresh thyme
½ tablespoon sage

1 tablespoon sea salt
½ teaspoon ground black pepper
¼ cup olive or avocado oil
8 boneless chicken breasts

Instructions:

1. Place all ingredients in a bag or storage container and let the chicken marinate for 2-24 hours.
2. Preheat grill on medium heat and grill chicken until cooked through but still moist (approximately 10 minutes on each side). Use extra marinade on chicken while cooking.

Optional: Can use marinade for vegetables as well.

Garnish with lemon wedges, rosemary sprigs, or Italian parsley.

Serves 8

Sweet Potato Pizza

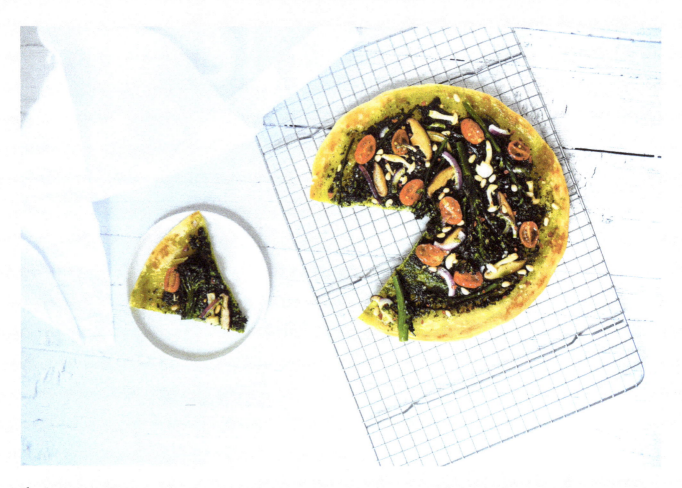

🍴 Ingredients:

Crust:
1 ½ cup white sweet potato, boiled and cooled (1 large or 2 small/medium)
½ cup arrowroot starch

¼ teaspoon sea salt
1 teaspoon olive oil

Pesto:
4 large cups basil

2 garlic cloves

1 handful or 1 cup spinach leaves
¾-1 cup olive oil

¼ cup pine nuts (omit if AIP)
Sea salt to taste

Sautéed Mushroom Topping:
1 tablespoon ghee
¼ cup Cremini mushrooms, sliced
¼ cup oyster or Shitake mushrooms, sliced
⅓ cup enoki mushrooms cut from the root
1 tablespoon roasted garlic, sliced in half
Sea salt and pepper to taste

Instructions:

Pesto:
Mix all ingredients in a mini chopper, blender, or food processor until well blended. Add more oil if needed.

Sautéed Mushroom Topping:
In a small pan on medium heat, melt ghee and add the mushrooms. Stir until cooked. Add sea salt and garlic and stir until combined.

Crust:
1. Preheat oven to 400 degrees.
2. Peel the potatoes, cut into chunks, and boil for 10 minutes or until soft. Drain and let cool.
3. In a food processor, place 1 ½ cups of sweet potato and blend for a minute until smooth. Add sea salt and arrowroot a little at a time and continue to blend until it starts to form a thick-like dough (about 2 minutes total). If it needs more arrowroot, add slowly.
4. On a baking sheet lined with parchment, spray or brush center with a bit of olive oil. Place dough evenly in a circular formation about an inch thick.
5. Lightly brush with olive oil in center to about an inch from the edge and place in the oven for 20-25 minutes or until edges begin to brown.
6. Turn the pizza crust over and bake for another 5-7 minutes.
7. Remove from oven and place pesto sauce and sautéed mushrooms in center.
8. Broil for 5-7 minutes.
9. Remove from oven and garnish with fresh cut basil and oregano.

Serves 2-4

PART II
THE FOODFRAME EATING LIFESTYLE

Before you jump into your new eating lifestyle, I want you to know that life is not perfect. Every meal might not be perfect; every day might not be perfect. My goal in writing this book is for everyone on this planet to eat more for survival and less for sport to maximize your health and quality of life. Aim as best as you can to stay in the healthy box most of the time. Of course, there will be celebrations, life events, and travel, or you may just feel like having that pizza or chips or chocolate cake, so you might decide to get out of the box. Don't worry—doing so is all part of life's experiences and joys. Take the opportunity to budget for those occasions and eat it if you really want it. Savor every morsel. Don't go crazy or go overboard but enjoy what you have budgeted for and get right back in the box. Do not wait for next Monday, or after your vacation, or an extended start time to change how you eat. This way, you can maintain your goals, your health, and your dignity.

I've found that so many people I work with will step out of the box for whatever reason and start having a running, negative conversation with themselves. Saying things like "I am bad," or "As long as I'm being bad, I might as well just keep eating what I want," or "I'm weak." I have a feeling you know what I'm talking about!

For some people, it can take months if not years, to get back into the box. In my office, my clients and I call it mental Vietnam--all the self-defeating things we say to ourselves after we've eaten something not on the program. Such as "Why did I do that?" or "I can't believe I did that," or "I can't ever be thin." Then we start making deals with ourselves like "I will do a double or longer workout tomorrow," or "I promise, I will never do this again," or "I won't attend the celebration dinner for my friend to make up for this." Sounds familiar? If so, that's because this is the exact time when people get tripped up, when you have that punitive conversation with yourself. They consider their new diet or eating plan an all-or-nothing deal, and when they fall off, they are *off*.

Instead, I want you to consider FoodFrame as a lifestyle. Like anything else new that you choose to incorporate into your life, it can take time to master—but when you stumble you know you should pick yourself up without judgment and keep living according to plan. It's *not* an all-or-nothing deal. I tell my clients that they will probably eat every day for the rest of their lives, so they have plenty of time to find balance. As long as most days are clean, you can be okay with the days—and the meals you eat--that aren't.

I don't believe in punishment because I know there is no such thing as perfect, and I've yet to meet anyone who eats a perfectly healthy diet all the time. The only difference, for me at least, between who I am and who I want to be…is what I *do*. This is what I tell my clients. Consistency *will* pay off for you. Whatever you tell yourself is probably true. So be kind to yourself and say nice things, and if you happen to get out of the box, well, you're only human. Just get right back in without judgment, punishment, or self-defeating conversations.

BEFORE YOU START

Remember: It is important to know these are not diets with the sole intention of helping you lose weight. These are *lifestyles* with the intention of optimizing your health with the side effect of weight loss. **What I tell people all the time is that you can eat whatever you want--you are just choosing to eat the foods that benefit you.** I really want you to remember that! Eating clean is the highest form of self-respect. Don't you deserve that?

- For all FoodFrames in the following chapters, you will find a detailed listing of foods to enjoy and those to avoid, as well as some of my favorite recipes for each diet. These will include a shake, soup, salad, appetizer or snack, entrée, side dish, and dessert.
- You are welcome to get creative in the kitchen or dine out using the food lists provided for each diet type. Every meal should include protein, fat, and fiber to keep you satiated and nourished. To make these FoodFrames easier to follow, there is no weighing and measuring of your food.

For protein: I generally recommend keeping animal proteins to the size of your palm, (except for Keto, and omit for vegetarian).

For vegetables: you can eat unlimited quantities any way you want them except for deep-fried or slathered in chemical or sugar-laden dressings or sauces.

For fats: always include a good-quality one.

- Trust your body. It knows what it needs and when it's had enough. Be conscious of your body when you are eating which will enable you to listen when it communicates with you. Eat when you're hungry and don't when you are not.
- Begin your Food Frame journey during a time when you know it will be easiest for you to follow it. For example, if you know you have a lot of business travel or family commitments coming up where you will not be able to control what you eat, you might want to wait until you know you can be in charge of your meal planning. Once you get going it will be easy to travel and go to social events as you will have the tools necessary to face these situations.

What to Do When You're Eating Out

We all dine out from time to time; some of us more than others. It's a part of life and it's important to find a balance. I always encourage people to cook at home as much as possible because you can have control over what ingredients are in your food, but if you know what to look out for, it's easier to navigate the dangers when you're in a restaurant. Here are some pointers:

- Most restaurants post their menus online. Take the time to look at the menu before agreeing to a restaurant, and make sure there will be an animal protein (or substitute, if you're a vegetarian or vegan), vegetables, and good fats available.

- Choose a restaurant that has minimally processed foods, bread, pasta, and heavy or creamy sauces.
- Tell the wait staff when you arrive about foods that you are unable to eat, such as gluten, dairy, or soy, for example.
- If you feel comfortable, ask what type of oil they use when cooking. Many restaurants, regardless of how nice they are, use highly processed vegetable or soybean oils which can quickly go rancid and cause inflammation. These oils won't kill you, but they cause their share of destruction and you really want to keep them to a minimum for optimal health, so it's always good to know which restaurants use them. And know that "crispy" is just another word for deep-fried!
- Stay away from the chips or bread that they bring to the table. If you arrive and are very hungry and find yourself tempted, ask the wait staff for fresh-cut vegetables or a salad right away. Or, you might want to have a small, healthy snack, like some nuts, a jerky stick, or a bit of hummus with cut-up veggies, before you arrive to take the edge off. You can always ask for a cup of herbal tea or lots of water with lemon as well before the meal comes or during dessert.
- If you know you are going to a restaurant or event that is going to be challenging, have a collagen protein shake before you go or on the way there. It will fill you up, so you won't be tempted to indulge, and you'll be able to enjoy the company of friends or family without distraction. I do this a lot and it works every time.

CHAPTER 4

THE PALEO FOODFRAME

The Paleo diet was originally created in the 1970s, but has since been referred to as the Caveman, Hunter-Gatherer, Stone Age, or Ancient diet. The reason for this is simple—this eating plan is based on the premise that humans will do best if they eat the way our ancestors ate to survive prior to the development of grain-centric modern agriculture. Loren Cordain, PhD, a scientist and former professor in the Department of Health and Exercise Science at Colorado State University, is one of the creators of the Paleo Diet. His belief is that people who lived during the Paleolithic Age (from 2.5 million to 10,000 years ago) mostly ate the wild animals they hunted and fished, along with native greens, roots, fruit, nuts, and seeds. Because the human body evolves very slowly, the Paleo diet is based on those same foods. Eating cleanly and simply—with foods that are anti-inflammatory in nature—helps you avoid modern-day health conditions caused by packaged and processed "fake" foods filled with chemicals, dyes, preservatives, and additives.

In the early 2000s, the Paleo diet became more popular among functional medicine followers, nutritionists, wellness professionals, and workout studios. CrossFit exercise studios were among one of the early adopters of Paleo as they touted it for weight loss, effective workout results, and optimal health to all their clients in conjunction with their workouts. Today, Paleo is quite common as it is easy to follow and promotes weight loss, and many additional diets have been formulated with a Paleo foundation.

With the Paleo FoodFrame, you will mainly be eating quality protein, fat, and fiber. This includes animal protein; unlimited vegetables cooked any way except fried; good fats that are mostly mono- or polyunsaturated fatty acids like avocado, olives, nuts, and high-quality oils; eggs; nuts and seeds; and yams or sweet potatoes. Due to the seasonality of fruit, it is included in moderation. In today's modern world we can get practically any fruit we want, virtually any time of the year, from just about every country that produces that fruit. In the Paleolithic era, humans were only able to eat fruit that was available in season, which was usually in the summertime, in order to gain weight to survive the winters. You'll be cutting back on fruit and only eating it in moderation to decrease your sugar levels—as you know by now, all fruits and carbs are converted to sugars in the body.

In addition, the Paleo FoodFrame focuses on quality, and unprocessed foods. Its premise is that modern-day farming and agriculture of legumes, grains, and dairy are not compatible for human DNA, so they are not permitted on the diet. All animal proteins should be grass-fed and grass-finished; seafood should be wild and not farmed; and poultry should be pastured or cage-free and organic. Produce should be organic as much as possible, and you can eat unlimited low-starchy vegetables, good fats, nuts and seeds.

WHAT PALEO IS BEST FOR

If I had to pick one eating plan that fits most people across the board, this would be the one. Most of my clients are either starting with Paleo after the RGN detox or maintaining on Paleo. It's especially beneficial for those with blood sugar issues and heart disease. Most people do well eating this way as it is easy to adhere to and convenient for traveling and dining out.

Critics of Paleo often refer to it as the "Meat diet," but it was never intended to be that way. It's not just about eating a lot of meat, and I don't recommend that anyone eat more meat or animal protein than their body actually needs. (See p. 17 for how to calculate your protein requirements.) Paleo should be a balanced eating plan, and your plate should be comprised of 60-80 percent vegetables, 15-20 percent animal protein, and 5-20 percent healthy fats.

The best thing about Paleo is that it can be maintained for a lifetime; you can stay on the Paleo FoodFrame indefinitely and continue to reap the benefits. It's not about counting calories but rather about putting the quality nourishment you need into your body. It more specifically helps with:

- **Reducing Systemic Inflammation.** Many of the foods consumed are anti-inflammatory in nature such as vegetables, nuts, seeds, and fruits. They contain high levels of fiber and antioxidants which assist in the elimination of harmful free radicals that contribute to inflammation. The Paleo FoodFrame is also high in omega-3 fatty acids sourced from fish, eggs, nuts, and oils that also help reduce inflammation.
- **Weight loss**. We know that sugar makes us fat. As a result, when you eat real food versus packaged and processed foods high in sugar and carbohydrates, you will lose weight. Realize, however, that weight loss can vary depending on what your weight was before you started on Paleo, along with other health and lifestyle factors. If, however, your weight is at or below normal levels, and you don't want to lose any weight, you should be able to maintain your ideal weight. Gaining weight can be achieved as well by increasing good carbohydrates and

protein if optimal absorption is present and your thyroid and blood sugars are regulated.
- **Regulating blood sugar**. When you stop eating sugar, grains, legumes, and processed foods that are all high in carbohydrates, you are automatically consuming less carbohydrates that convert straight into sugar. In addition, this FoodFrame includes quality protein and fats which are digested slowly to support balanced levels of blood sugar.
- **Reducing high blood pressure**. Eating in a way that replaces sugar or grains with nutrient-dense foods filled with vitamins, minerals, and antioxidants contributes to lower hypertension levels.
- **Supporting Cardiovascular Health**. It is a well-established fact that heart disease is correlated to a diet high in sugar and processed foods. By removing those "junk" foods, you should see an improvement in your cholesterol and triglyceride levels, blood pressure, body fat, Type 2 diabetes, and insulin resistance.
- **Alzheimer's Disease**. Due to reduced blood sugar, the Paleo diet can reduce symptoms and slow down its progression.
- **Acne**. Lower insulin levels and eating less sugar, processed foods, and gluten can help improve acne and the appearance of your skin. Increased insulin and androgens, the male hormones made in the adrenal glands, are a major contributor to acne. In addition, many people will get acne from gluten and dairy.
- **Improving Energy**. You should experience more energy and enhanced mental focus due to support from your mitochondria, which produces the energy in your cells.

SIDEBAR – Nancy's Story

Nancy, age 51, came into my office feeling horrible. Her primary complaint was joint pain all over her body, but that was concentrated mostly in her knees, shoulders, and elbows. This was a huge problem for her as she was a longtime kindergarten teacher and needed to get up and down off the floor with the kids throughout the day. In tears, she told me she could no longer sit cross-legged on the floor or go up and down the stairs in her home other than to get to bed and leave the house. She also experienced daily fatigue, chronic weekly headaches, and hot flashes. After being told she had Graves Disease, she'd twice had radiation treatments on her thyroid.

Nancy's diet consisted of a small variety of mostly processed foods, and she rarely ate vegetables. Because she didn't like to cook, she usually grabbed food for convenience rather than for her health. She wanted to lose weight and feel better.

I put her on the RGN Detox and within two weeks her joint pain had substantially decreased. She begged me to continue the detox which I agreed to, and twenty-eight days later she was practically a new person. We kept her on a Paleo FoodFrame containing animal protein, vegetables, good fats, sweet potatoes, and yams. Removing legumes, grains, alcohol, and sugar made all the difference in the world. I also ordered a stool test and found that Nancy had a significant amount of a bacteria called Prevotella Copri, a pre-curser to rheumatoid arthritis—a condition her mother had struggled with for many years. We treated the bacteria naturally with anti-bacterial and anti-microbial supplements.

Nancy lost a total of 45 pounds and fit into the shorts she wore on her honeymoon, which she was able to wear when she and her husband went on a trip to celebrate their thirtieth wedding anniversary. She continues to eat a Paleo FoodFrame with one to two collagen shakes per day.

WHO SHOULD AVOID PALEO

Anyone can do this FoodFrame, no matter what their age or health condition. Vegetarians and vegans can also follow this eating plan with modified amounts of legumes as their protein source along with nuts and seeds. They are often referred to as Pegans.

PALEO FOODS TO ENJOY

Meat

Includes broth and collagen

Cattle (beef, veal), deer (venison), goat, hare, pig (pork), rabbit, sheep (lamb, mutton), wild game (buffalo/bison, boar, elk)

Poultry

Includes broth and collagen

Chicken, duck, goose, grouse, hen, ostrich, pheasant, quail, turkey

Fish

Includes broth and collagen

Anchovy, arctic char, bass, bonito, carp, catfish, cod, eel, gar, haddock, hake, halibut, herring, mackerel, mahi-mahi, marlin, monkfish, perch, pollock, salmon, sardine, snapper, sole, swordfish, tilapia, trout, tuna, ahi, yellowfin, turbot, walleye

Shellfish

Includes broth and collagen

Clams, crab, crawfish, lobster, mussels, octopus, oysters, scallops, shrimp, squid

Eggs

Chicken, duck, goose, quail, including fish eggs/caviar

Leafy Vegetables

Unlimited

Arugula, beet greens, Bok choy, broccoli rabe, Brussels sprouts, cabbage, carrot tops, celery, chicory, collard greens, cress, dandelion greens, endive, all varieties of kale, all varieties of lettuces, mustard greens, Napa cabbage, purslane, radicchio, sorrel, spinach, swiss chard, tatsoi, turnip greens, watercress

Non-starchy Vegetables

Artichoke, asparagus, broccoli, cauliflower, celery, fennel, rhubarb, squash blossoms

Allium-family Vegetables

Chive, garlic, leek, onion, scallion, shallot, wild leek

Roots, Tubers, and Bulb Vegetables

Arrowroot, bamboo shoot, beet, burdock, carrot, cassava, celeriac, daikon, ginger, horseradish, Jerusalem artichoke, jicama, kohlrabi, lotus root, parsnip, radish, rutabaga, sweet potato, taro, turnip, wasabi, water chestnut, yam

Nightshades or Spices Derived from Nightshades

Omit or limit if Autoimmune (see Chapter 5)

Ashwagandha, capsicums/peppers, chili pepper flakes, chili powder, curry, cayenne pepper, paprika, pepinos, peppers (bell, chipotle, hot, red, and sweet), and pimentos; cape gooseberries, eggplant, goji berries (wolfberries), potatoes (sweet potatoes and yams are not nightshades and are okay), sweet plantains, tomatoes (all varieties)

Sea Vegetables

Arame, dulse, hijiki, kombu, nori, wakame

Vegetable-like Fruits

Avocado, bitter melon, chayote, cucumber, okra, olives, plantain, pumpkin, squash, winter melon, zucchini

Berries

0-1 serving daily

Acai, blackberry, blueberry, cranberry, currant, elderberry, gooseberry, grapes (all varieties), lingonberry, mulberry, raspberry, strawberry

Rosaceae-family Fruits

In moderation

Apple, apricot, cherry, nectarine, peach, pear, plum, quince, rosehip

Melons

In moderation

Cantaloupe, honeydew, horned melon, melon pear, Persian melon, watermelon, winter melon

Citrus-family Fruits

In moderation

Clementine, grapefruit, kumquat, lemon, lime, orange, pomelo, tangelo, tangerine, yuzu

Tropical fruits

In moderation

Acerola, banana, chayote, cherimoya, coconut, date, dragon fruit, durian, fig, guava, jackfruit, kiwi, loquat, lychee, mango, mangosteen, papaya, passion fruit, pawpaw, persimmon, pineapple, plantain, pomegranate, star fruit, tamarind

Edible Fungi/Mushrooms

Chanterelle, cremini, morel, oyster, porcini, portobello, shiitake, truffle

Animal Fats

Bacon fat, ghee, lard, leaf lard (fat from pig), pan drippings, poultry fat, chicken or goose fat, strutto (clarified pork fat), tallow (from beef, lamb, or mutton)

Plant Fats

Avocado oil (cold-pressed), coconut oil, extra virgin olive oil (cold-pressed), flaxseed oil, palm oil, palm shortening, sesame oil, walnut oil

Nuts/Nut Butters and Nut Oils

Almonds, Brazil nuts, cashews, chestnuts, hazelnuts, macadamia, pistachios, pecans, pine nuts, walnuts

Seeds and Seed Oils

Chia, flax, hemp, poppy, pumpkin, sesame, sunflower

Probiotic Foods

Fermented meat or fish, kombucha, kvass, lacto-fermented fruits and vegetables, non-dairy kefir, sauerkraut

Herbs and Spices

Allspice, anise, annatto, basil leaf, bay leaf, black caraway, cardamom, celery seed, chamomile, Chinese five-spice powder, chervil, chives, cilantro, coriander, cinnamon, cloves, cumin, curry powder, dill, fennel seed, fennel leaf, fenugreek, garlic, ginger, garam masala, juniper, kaffir lime leaf, lavender, lemongrass, mace, marjoram leaf, mustard, nutmeg, onion powder, oregano leaf, parsley, pepper, peppermint, poppy, rosemary, saffron, sage, savory leaf, sea or Himalayan salt, spearmint, tarragon, thyme, truffles, turmeric, vanilla

Flavorings

Watch for added ingredients

Anchovies or anchovy paste, apple cider vinegar, balsamic vinegar, capers, carob powder, coconut aminos (a soy sauce substitute), coconut concentrate, coconut milk, coconut water vinegar, fish sauce, fruit and vegetable juices (in moderation), organic jams and chutneys (in moderation), red wine vinegar, truffle oil (made with olive oil), white wine vinegar

Sweeteners

In moderation

Allulose, coconut sugar, coconut syrup, erythritol, lucuma, maple sugar, maple syrup, molasses, monk fruit (Luo Han Guo), raw honey, stevia; trace amounts of cane sugar are okay in cured meats and kombucha

Beverages

Water (club, mineral, reverse osmosis, seltzer, soda, sparkling [without natural flavors, sweeteners, or additives], spring); almond milk (unsweetened), coconut water (in moderation), coconut milk, hemp milk (unsweetened), herbal teas

Foods Included in Moderation

Fructose (less than 10–20 grams per day), green or black tea, moderate to high glycemic load fruits/vegetables (dried fruit, plantain, taro, etc.), omega-6 polyunsaturated fat-rich foods (poultry and industrially raised fatty meat), yerba mate

PALEO - FOODS TO AVOID

Grains and Grain-Like Foods

Amaranth, barley, buckwheat, bulgur, corn, farro, millet, oats/oatmeal, quinoa, rice, wild rice, rye, sorghum, spelt, teff, wheat (all varieties, including einkorn and semolina)

Dairy

Butter, buttermilk, cheese (all types), cream (all varieties), curds, dairy-protein isolates, ice cream, kefir, milk, whey, whey-protein isolate, yogurt

Legumes

Adzuki beans, black beans, black-eyed peas, butter beans, calico beans, cannellini beans, chickpeas (garbanzo beans), fava beans (broad beans), great northern beans, green beans, Italian beans, kidney beans, lentils, lima beans, mung beans, navy beans, peanuts, peas, pinto beans, runner beans, soybeans (including edamame, tofu, tempeh, other soy products, and soy isolates, such as soy lecithin), split peas

Processed Vegetable Oils

Canola oil (rapeseed oil), corn oil, cottonseed oil, grapeseed oil, palm kernel oil, peanut oil, safflower oil, soybean oil, sunflower oil

Processed Food Chemicals and Ingredients

Acrylamides, any ingredient with an unrecognizable chemical name, artificial and natural flavors, artificial food color, autolyzed protein, brominated vegetable oil, emulsifiers (carrageenan, cellulose gum, guar gum, lecithin), hydrolyzed vegetable protein, monosodium glutamate, nitrates or nitrites (naturally occurring are okay), olestra, phosphoric acid, propylene glycol, textured vegetable protein, trans fats (partially hydrogenated vegetable oil, hydrogenated oil), yeast extract

Sugars

Agave, agave nectar, barley malt, barley malt syrup, beet sugar, brown rice syrup, brown sugar, cane crystals, cane juice, cane sugar, raw cane sugar, evaporated cane juice, and dehydrated cane juice, caramel, corn sweetener, corn syrup, and corn syrup solids, crystalline fructose, date sugar, demerara sugar, dextrin, dextrose, fructose, high-fructose corn syrup, fruit juice, fruit juice concentrate, glucose, glucose solids, golden syrup, invert sugar, jaggery, lactose, malt syrup, maltodextrin, maltose, muscovado sugar, palm sugar, raw sugar, refined sugar, rice bran syrup, rice syrup, saccharose, sorghum syrup, sucanat, sucrose, syrup, treacle, turbinado sugar, yacon syrup

Sugar Alcohols

Naturally occurring sugar alcohols found in whole foods like fruit are okay.

Malitol, mannitol, sorbitol, xylitol

Non-nutritive Sweeteners

Acesulfame potassium, aspartame (Sweet 'n Low, Equal), neotame, saccharin, sucralose (Splenda)

Nuts and Nut Oils

Peanuts and peanut oil

Alcohol

Alcoholic beverages are technically not permitted (small amounts in kombucha are okay) on Paleo. However, some choose to have alcohol in moderation; the best choices are distilled liquors like vodka, tequila, or gin as they contain minimal processing and the lowest sugar content. Recommended with sparkling water and lemon or lime.

Beverages

Coffee (decaf and caffeinated), cow milk, dairy-based kefir, electrolyte drinks, energy drinks, fruit juices, rice milk, sodas (diet and regular), soymilk, sports drinks; any drinks containing artificial coloring, flavors, sweeteners, or preservatives.

PALEO - RECIPES

Golden Milk

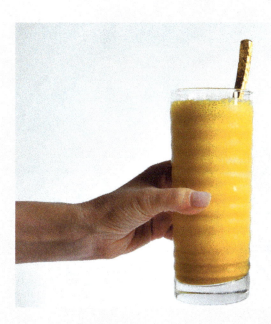

🍴 Ingredients:

2 cups unsweetened full fat coconut milk
2 scoops RGN Collagen Protein, vanilla
2 tablespoons coconut oil
1 teaspoon ground turmeric

½ teaspoon ground cinnamon
¼ teaspoon ground ginger
Pinch of black pepper
1 tablespoon honey, optional

🍴 Instructions:

1. Place all ingredients into a saucepan and heat while stirring until fully combined.

Serve warm.

Note: You can use fresh turmeric and ginger root, just strain after cooking.

Serves 2

Paleo Hash

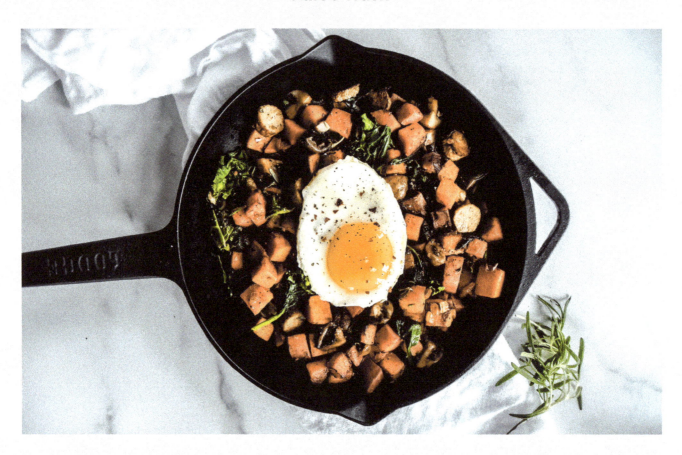

🍴 Ingredients:

2 tablespoons ghee or coconut oil
1 medium yam, washed, with skin and cubed
½ cup red or yellow onion, diced
½ cup button mushrooms, quartered
3 chicken sausages (nitrite and nitrate-free), sliced into rounds
1 handful red kale, washed, stems removed, and cut into pieces
1 handful spinach
1 teaspoon chopped rosemary
1 teaspoon thyme
Sea salt and pepper to taste

🍴 Instructions:

1. In an iron skillet melt ghee or coconut oil and add cubed yam.
2. Stir until soft and slightly brown. Add sausages, mushrooms, and onions. Continue to stir until sausages are cooked.
3. Add kale, spinach, and herbs. Cook until greens are wilted.

Serve with or without a fried egg on top.

Serves 2-4

Paleo Chili

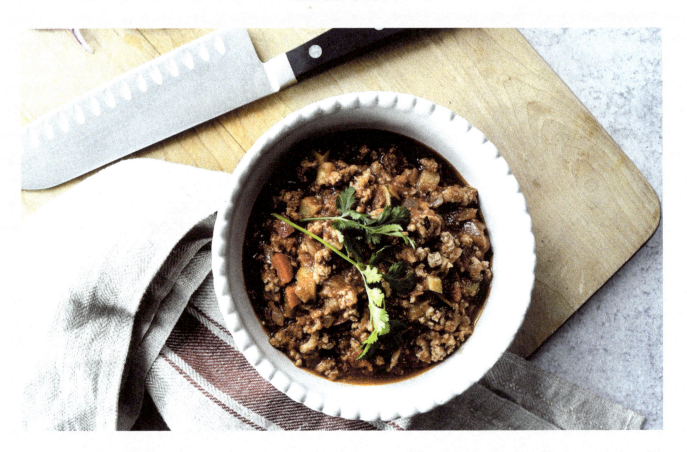

🍴 Ingredients:

1 tablespoon coconut oil
1 white onion, chopped
1 organic yellow pepper, diced
1 organic red pepper, diced
1 large organic zucchini, diced
1 Jalapeno, diced (keep some of the seeds if you want it spicy) and more for garnish
1 28 oz. can organic peeled and diced tomatoes
Diced red onion, jalapeno slices, and avocado for garnish

2 tablespoons organic tomato paste
3 teaspoons cumin
½ teaspoon chili powder
¼ teaspoon cayenne
Sea salt and pepper to taste
2 pounds of grass-fed and finished beef (or ground chicken or turkey, dark meat)

Instructions:

1. In a soup pot, melt coconut oil. Add onion, red and yellow peppers, zucchini, and jalapeno. Cook until soft. Add cumin, chili powder, and cayenne and mix until combined.
2. Add beef and break apart to remove all clumps. Stir until the meat is cooked.
3. Drain tomato juice from the can and add tomatoes and tomato paste. Add sea salt and pepper to taste. Cook on low for another 20 minutes.

Garnish with chopped onions, jalapenos, and avocados.

Serves 4-6

Roasted Cauliflower

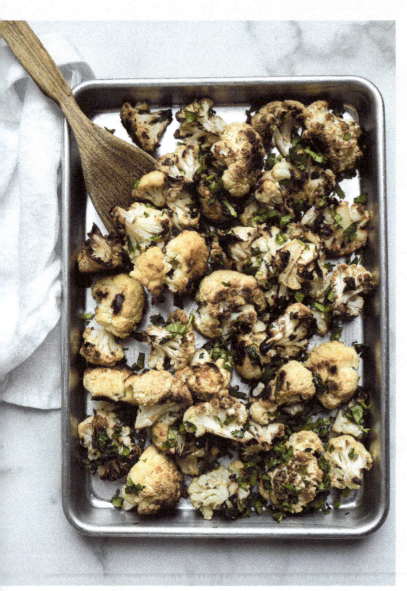

🧪 Ingredients:

2 heads cauliflower, trimmed
3-5 cloves garlic, minced
1-3 tablespoons olive oil
½-1 cup cilantro, chopped
Sea salt, to taste

🧪 Instructions:

Preheat oven to 400 degrees.
Preheat oven to 400 degrees.

1. Cut 2 heads of cauliflower into florets and place in a large bowl. Add minced garlic cloves and drizzle olive oil and toss to lightly coat. There should be no oil in the bottom of the bowl.
2. Place the cauliflower mixture on a cookie sheet and sprinkle with sea salt. Place in the preheated oven and cook until the bottoms have browned (about 20-25 minutes), then turn and cook for another 20-25 minutes.
3. Remove from the oven and place in a bowl. Mix in chopped cilantro, add a touch of salt if needed, and serve.

Serves 6-8

French Onion Soup

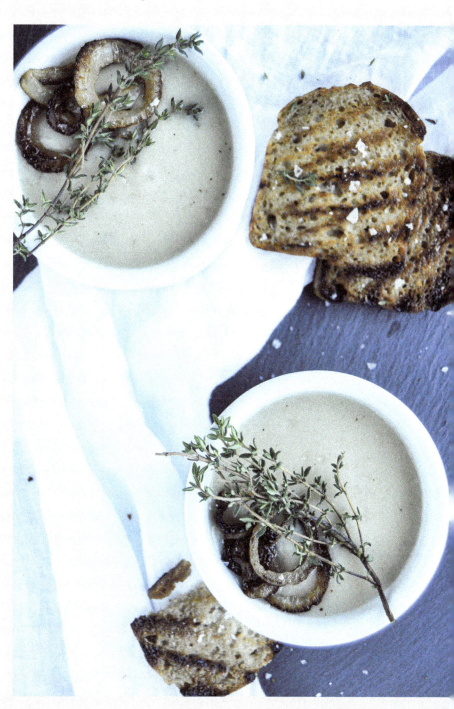

🍴 Ingredients:

6 tablespoons coconut oil or ghee
4 organic yellow onions, thinly sliced
1 tablespoon raw/local honey
3 garlic cloves, pressed or minced
¼ cup apple cider vinegar
7 cups vegetable or chicken broth
1 tablespoon sea salt
¼ teaspoon fresh thyme
2 bay leaves

🍴 Instructions:

Heat oil in a large pot over medium-high heat. Stir in onions until translucent. Add honey and reduce heat to medium. Stir onions occasionally and allow to cook for another 30 minutes.

Add garlic and apple cider vinegar. Cook on low for 2-4 hours.

Blend until smooth using a handheld/immersion blender, blender, or food processor and serve.

Serves 6-8

Grilled Chicken Salad with Mint Lime Dressing

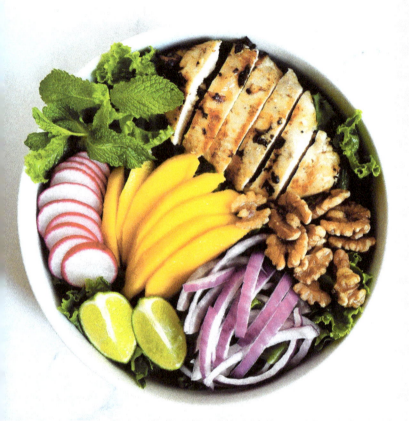

Ingredients:
4 boneless pastured chicken breasts

Marinade:
3 tablespoons lime juice
1 tablespoon minced garlic
¼ cup fresh mint leaves, chopped
⅓ cup avocado oil

Dressing:
1 ½ limes, juiced
½ cup olive oil
2 garlic cloves, minced
¼ cup fresh mint leaves, chopped
¼ cup raw or roasted walnuts
Pinch sea salt and pepper

Salad:
6 cups green leaf lettuce (any kind)
¼ cup radishes, sliced thinly
¼ cup mango, cut in thin julienne strips
¼ red onion, sliced thinly

Instructions:
1. In a glass container, combine chicken breasts with marinade and refrigerate for 4-24 hours.
2. On an indoor grill pan or outdoor grill, cook chicken with marinade until fully cooked.
3. While the chicken is cooking, assemble the salad and dressing.
4. Slice cooked chicken and place on top of salad. Drizzle with dressing.

Garnish with fresh mint.

Serves 4

Dark Chocolate Nut Squares

Ingredients:

1 ¼ cups unsalted roasted almonds, lightly chopped
½ cup unsalted roasted hazelnuts, lightly chopped
½ cup unsalted roasted pistachios, shelled
⅓ cup unsalted roasted sunflower seeds
7 oz dark chocolate, 72-90 percent cacao
⅓ cup coconut oil
½ cup monk fruit or stevia
½ teaspoon fine sea salt

Instructions:

Line a square 8" X 8" pan with parchment paper and set aside.

1. Place all chopped nuts and seeds in a bowl and mix until well combined.
2. In a double boiler, slowly melt the chocolate until smooth. Add coconut oil and stir until fully melted and well combined. Remove from heat and add monk fruit and sea salt. Stir to combine.
3. Pour the chocolate over the nuts and seeds in the bowl and stir until fully incorporated.
4. Place the chocolate-covered mixture in the parchment-lined pan and smooth out until evenly distributed. Place in the freezer for 30 minutes or more.
5. Remove from freezer and cut into small squares.

Store in the refrigerator in a tightly covered container.

Makes 16-20 bars

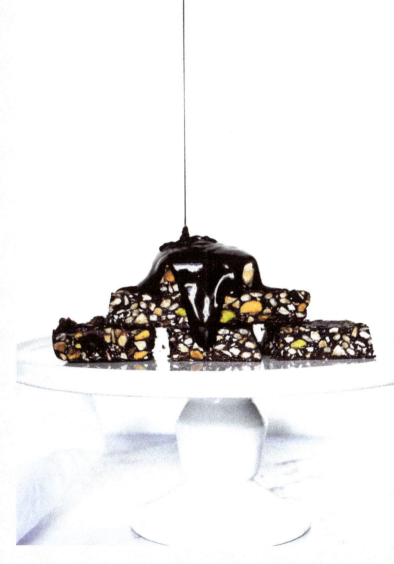

CHAPTER 5

THE KETOGENIC (KETO) FOODFRAME

Do you remember the South Beach diet or the Atkins diet? Or have you just read about Paleo in the previous chapter, and your interest is piqued? Well, these eating plans are all based on the premise of high-protein and low-carbohydrate meals. Some of those eating plans will have much higher levels of fats or dairy than you might be used to, while the Ketogenic (or Keto) FoodFrame consists of a very low-carbohydrate, high-fat eating style that includes grass-fed or wild animal protein, dairy, and many non-starchy vegetables. Do you love your butter and eggs? You can enjoy them when you eat the Keto way.

You might be surprised to learn that the Keto diet has been around for almost 100 years, as it was originally developed to treat drug-resistant epilepsy, especially in children. Dr. Robert Atkins popularized it in the 1970s for weight loss, but it fell out of favor before resurging again in 2018 as more science emerged with data showing the health benefits of Keto over time. As a result, I believe that Keto will continue to be popular as well as be helpful for the foreseeable future.

ABOUT KETOSIS

Carbohydrates fuel your body. Whenever we eat any food that contains sugars, whether it's fruit, sweets, dairy, or the carbohydrates that are found in bread, grains, legumes, or potatoes, your pancreas excretes insulin, the hormone responsible for managing your blood sugar levels. That insulin then converts the glucose into glycogen….which is then sent to your brain and every cell to create ATP…which is the energy that fuels every cell in your body. This is your body's fuel production process.

So, what would happen if you decided to provide your body with only very low levels of glucose? It would resort to using either your stored fat or newly consumed sources of fat (avocados, salmon, coconut) for energy rather than carbohydrates. In other words, the Keto FoodFrame switches the fuel source from carbohydrates (or anything that turns into sugar) to fat. As your body burns this fat, your liver breaks it down into fatty acids and glycerol in a process known as beta-oxidation. There are three primary types of ketone bodies made in the liver: acetoacetate, beta-hydroxybutyrate, and acetone. Once the ketone levels in the blood rise to a certain point, you enter into the metabolic state of ketosis.

The goal of ketosis is to stay fueled by circulating the energy-laden ketones—this is what burns the fat and leads to weight loss. You do this by sticking to this eating plan, with the following daily caloric percentages:

- Fat: 70-80 percent
- Animal Protein: 15-25 percent
- Carbohydrates: 5 percent or less
- Non-starchy vegetables: Unlimited to a degree

Typically, I do not recommend a large amount of animal protein to anyone—but Keto is the one exception. This really is the "meat diet" as animal protein and oils are the only two food groups that do not contain any carbohydrates but do contain fat, which is ideal here. With Keto, animal protein is basically unlimited, but I urge you to have a balanced eating plan with a variety of green and colored vegetables to maintain the protein, fat, and fiber levels you need. I always recommend moderation with animal protein as the consequences of excessive consumption often led to constipation. In addition, eating a lot of foods high in protein can cause strain on the kidneys.

Health Benefits of Ketosis

There are significant health benefits to ketosis.

- **Weight loss**. One study found that people on Keto lost 2.2 times more weight than those on a calorie-restricted low-fat diet. The ketones suppress ghrelin, the hunger hormone.
- **Improved blood sugar**. Studies have shown Keto to boost insulin sensitivity and fat loss, which leads to an improvement for Type 2 diabetes and pre-diabetes.
- **Heart disease**. Keto can lessen risk factors like body fat, triglycerides, HDL cholesterol, and high blood pressure.
- **Alzheimer's disease**. Due to reduced blood sugar, Keto can reduce symptoms and slow down its progression.
- **Acne**. Lower insulin levels and eating less sugar, processed foods, and gluten can help improve acne and the appearance of your skin. Increased insulin and androgens, the male hormones made in the adrenal glands, are a major contributor to acne. In addition, many people will get acne from gluten and dairy.
- **Improved energy**. You should experience more energy and enhanced mental focus due to the effective mitochondrial, which produce the energy in your cells.
- **Fuels the brain**. The human brain is comprised of 50-60 percent fat. Keto fat will keep the brain strong and functioning optimally.

Sticking to Ketosis

Following a Keto FoodFrame isn't difficult, but it takes some discipline--and consistency is key. Here is the challenge. You need to stick to an extreme minimizing of your carbohydrate and sugar intake, so you cut off your normal supply of glucose to your cells for energy. Eating enough fat and limiting carbohydrates is an absolute must. Once you get out of ketosis, it can take a few days to get back in, so even going off it with a bite here or there can really set you back.

For best results with weight loss and reducing blood sugar, aim to eat 20 grams of net carbs at the very most each day. Net carbs are calculated by total grams of carbohydrates minus dietary fiber. If sugar alcohols are on a label you subtract them as well for total net carbs. For example, one-half cup of raw almonds contains 14 grams of total carbohydrates and 8 grams of dietary fiber. Therefore, total net carbs are 6 grams. From my experience, those who have the best weight-loss results on Keto are strict when sticking to net carbs no higher than 20 grams per day. I recommend getting an app, like the Carb Manager, on your phone or on your computer to track your daily carb intake. You'll likely be surprised how quickly they can add up. Vegetables and nuts contain carbohydrates, too, so you need to track them carefully as every little bite counts.

The best way to know if you are in ketosis is to measure the ketones your body produces. You can easily do this by breath or urine testing when you first wake up each morning. These tests can be found online or even at health food stores. Also, be sure to drink half your body weight in ounces of water each day. Increase your potassium intake from leafy greens and avocados. Exercise can help you get into ketosis quicker, but don't overdo it.

At this point, you may be wondering how all this fat affects your cardiovascular health. Dr. Eric Westman, board-certified in Obesity Medicine and Internal Medicine, founded the Duke Lifestyle Medicine Clinic after eight years of clinical research on low carbohydrate and ketogenic diets. According to the science Dr. Westman studied regarding the safety of Keto, one of the causes of heart disease is metabolic syndrome, which develops when a person has elevated triglycerides, low levels of HDL (High Density Lipoprotein, also known as the "good" cholesterol), excess weight carried in the mid-section, elevated blood pressure, and elevated blood glucose, which basically translates into insulin resistance. His research found that Keto is helpful in weight loss and stabilizing blood sugar, which affects triglycerides and blood pressure; the metabolic syndrome improves and, consequently, so does heart disease.[5]

---

[5] https://www.adaptyourlife.com/dr-eric-westman/top-4-benefits-of-low-carb-or-keto/

Treating metabolic syndrome: There's a new understanding that metabolic syndrome is the cause of heart disease and atherosclerosis or hardening of the arteries. If you have high triglyceride and low HDL (good cholesterol), elevated blood sugar that isn't full-blown diabetes, and elevated blood pressure that's not quite high blood pressure, this is called metabolic syndrome. To determine if you have it, you'll need to have tests done by your doctor.

Cholesterol is neither the enemy nor a golf score. You need cholesterol for many different bodily functions; without it, you can't produce hormones or vitamin D, which helps make calcium. Cholesterol also plays the role of messenger as it transports other vitamins into your bones. It is also essential for building tissue and helps the liver produce bile. Basically, you don't want your cholesterol numbers to go too low. Additionally, many studies have shown that the old science of high cholesterol levels, specifically LDL (Low Density Lipoprotein, also known as the "bad" cholesterol) does not automatically equate to heart disease. Other factors that contribute to heart disease are exercise, smoking, alcohol consumption, and lifestyle factors such as stress, happiness, and quality of relationships.

KETO IS BEST FOR

Those who are obese or overweight and need or want to lose weight and have no health issues preventing them from trying this FoodFrame, should seriously consider it. If you follow it carefully, you *will* lose weight. Keto also gives people more energy and mental focus (as I said earlier in this chapter, your brain is 50-60 % fat!). In addition, anyone with Polycystic Ovarian Syndrome (PCOS) or cancer of any kind, either currently or previously, would benefit greatly from Keto, as scientists have discovered that sugar feeds cancer cells.[6]

I recommend Keto for people with substantial blood sugar dysregulation such as pre-diabetes, diabetes, or insulin resistance. Because it completely removes sugar and severely limits foods that turn into sugar, it can be highly effective and expeditious in balancing blood sugars. Keto is also recommended for pediatric epilepsy as high fat levels have been shown to reduce the frequency of epileptic seizures. In addition, many of my clients have told me that they are not as hungry on Keto as they were on other eating plans, no doubt because they're eating more fat and proteins, foods which are satiating over longer periods of time.

SIDEBAR – Jan's Story

---

[6] https://www.mdanderson.org/publications/focused-on-health/FOH-cancer-love-sugar.h14-1589835.html
"It's true that sugar feeds every cell in our body — even cancer cells. But, research shows that eating sugar doesn't necessarily lead to cancer. It's what sugar does to your waistline that can lead to cancer."
https://www.nature.com/articles/s41467-017-01019-z
Yeast and cancer cells share the unusual characteristic of favoring fermentation of sugar over respiration. We now reveal an evolutionary conserved mechanism linking fermentation to activation of Ras, a major regulator of cell proliferation in yeast and mammalian cells, and prime proto-oncogene product. A yeast mutant (*tps1Δ*) with overactive influx of glucose into glycolysis and hyperaccumulation of Fru1,6bisP, shows hyperactivation of Ras, which causes its glucose growth defect by triggering apoptosis.

Jan called my office in a bit of a panic. Her hair had suddenly started falling out in huge clumps, which had created bald spots on her scalp. Her doctor confirmed it was not alopecia but left her without a plan to heal. In addition, she discovered dryness and redness around her neck and ears and was also suffering from diarrhea three times a week, monthly headaches, and chronic soreness in her right calf.

After ordering blood and stool tests, I immediately put her on the RGN Detox to clean out the system and optimize her liver function, which brought her relief from the diarrhea, headaches, and calf pain. Once we found out she had the gene mutation MTHFR, I gave her the correct amounts of B vitamins along with support for her adrenal glands and put her on a Paleo FoodFrame. Her hair started to grow back, and all the other symptoms disappeared.

Because Jan admitted she was about 90 % compliant--she was holding onto her nightly glass of wine for dear life—she lost 12 pounds but could not lose any of the 10 more pounds she wanted to drop. I ordered follow-up blood tests and found active Epstein-Barr virus and Cytomegalovirus. We treated those naturally and I switched her to a Keto FoodFrame. At this stage, Keto was the best choice because her weight loss had plateaued on Paleo; she was more efficient at burning fat when fueled with fat rather than carbohydrates. In addition, she had some blood sugar dysregulation which Keto is effective at stabilizing.

After only one week on the Keto diet, Jan felt amazing and started to lose the weight. She stayed on it for two months until her blood sugars normalized, and she was able to maintain her goal weight. She told me that when she puts her hair in a ponytail now, she can tell how much thicker her hair is. She'd given up hope that it would ever grow back!

WHO SHOULD AVOID KETO

Keto is a fairly restrictive way to eat, and I've found that many clients do much better when it's used for the short-term, two to three months, but it has been proven safe to follow Keto long-term if you can stick to it scrupulously. Although I must add that Paleo is much easier to sustain for a lifetime of good health.

As for weight loss, most men do very well with Keto, but not quite as many women, especially those with adrenal issues, such as a cortisol imbalance or chronic, high level stress. Women will lose weight but some not as much as others. It is not recommended for people without a gallbladder, kidney issues, or who have trouble metabolizing fats.

Also, since you mostly eat animal protein on the Keto diet, it is exceedingly difficult for a vegan to follow it. The inclusion of dairy makes it easier for vegetarians to follow, but not vegans, and some may still find it challenging.

The Keto Flu

At the onset of the Keto FoodFrame, some people come down with what's referred to as the Keto Flu, a collection of flu-like symptoms that vary in severity and can include:

- Bad breath
- Bloating
- Constipation
- Diarrhea
- Dizziness
- Fatigue
- Increased cravings
- Moodiness or irritability
- Muscle cramps or soreness
- Nausea
- Sleep disturbance
- Stomach pain
- Vomiting

These symptoms are caused by the switch of your energy source from carbs to fat. They are *all temporary* and should go away within three days to two weeks. It usually affects those who are used to eating a lot of carbs or a highly processed diet before they go Keto; if you already eat a low-carb diet, most likely you will not get this "flu."

To decrease any symptoms, stay hydrated, avoid strenuous exercise, use quality sea salt, eat plenty of green leafy vegetables and avocados as they are high in potassium to ensure proper electrolyte balance, and get plenty of sleep.

KETO FOODS TO ENJOY

Meat

Includes broth and collagen

Cattle (beef, veal), deer (venison), goat, hare, pig (pork), rabbit, sheep (lamb, mutton), wild game (buffalo/bison, boar, elk)

Poultry

Includes broth and collagen

Chicken, duck, goose, grouse, hen, ostrich, pheasant, quail, turkey

Fish

Includes broth and collagen

Anchovy, arctic char, bass, bonito, carp, catfish, cod, eel, gar, haddock, hake, halibut, herring, mackerel, mahi-mahi, marlin, monkfish, perch, pollock, salmon, sardine, snapper, sole, swordfish, tilapia, trout, tuna, ahi, yellowfin, turbot, walleye

Shellfish

Clams, crab, crawfish, lobster, mussels, octopus, oysters, scallops, shrimp, squid

Eggs

Chicken, duck, goose, quail, including fish eggs/caviar

Dairy

Butter, buttermilk, cheese (all types), cream (all varieties), dairy-protein isolates, ghee, kefir, milk, curds, all varieties of whey, low carb/low sugar yogurt (in moderation)

Leafy Vegetables

*In moderation

Arugula, beet greens, Bok choy, broccoli rabe, Brussels sprouts, cabbage, carrot tops, celery, chicory, collard greens, cress, dandelion greens, endive, kale, all varieties, lettuce, all varieties, mustard greens, Napa cabbage, purslane, radicchio, sorrel, spinach, swiss chard, tatsoi, turnip greens, watercress

Non-starchy Vegetables

*In moderation

Artichoke, asparagus, broccoli, cauliflower, celery, fennel, rhubarb (stems only), squash blossoms

Allium-family Vegetables

Chive, garlic, leek, onion, scallion, shallot, wild leek

Roots, Tubers, and Bulb Vegetables

*In moderation

Arrowroot, bamboo shoot, beet, burdock, carrot, celeriac, daikon, ginger, horseradish and root, Jerusalem artichoke, jicama, kohlrabi, lotus root, parsnip, radish, rutabaga, turnip, wasabi, water chestnut, yam noodles

Sea Vegetables

Arame, dulse, hijiki, kombu, nori, wakame

Vegetable-like Fruits

Avocado, cucumber, olives

Edible Fungi/Mushrooms

Chanterelle, cremini, morel, oyster, porcini, portobello, shiitake, truffle

Animal Fats

Bacon fat, lard, leaf lard (fat from a pig), pan drippings, poultry fat, schmaltz (chicken or goose fat), strutto (clarified pork fat), tallow (from beef, lamb, or mutton)

Plant Fats

Avocado oil (cold-pressed), coconut oil, extra virgin olive oil (cold-pressed), palm oil, palm shortening, red palm oil, sesame oil

Processed Vegetable Oils

*Permitted but not recommended

Canola oil (rapeseed oil), corn oil, cottonseed oil, grapeseed oil, palm kernel oil, peanut oil, safflower oil, soybean oil, sunflower oil

Citrus Family Fruits

Lemon, lime

Probiotic Foods

Fermented meat or fish, kombucha, kvass, lacto-fermented vegetables, non-dairy kefir, sauerkraut

Non-nutritive Sweeteners

Permitted but not recommended

Acesulfame potassium, aspartame (Sweet 'n Low, Equal), neotame, saccharin, sucralose (Splenda)

Nuts, Nut Oils, and Nut Butters

In moderation

Almonds, brazil nuts, cashews, chestnuts, hazelnuts, macadamia, peanuts, pecans, pine nuts, pistachios, walnuts

Seeds and Seed Butter

In moderation

Chia, flax, hemp, poppy, pumpkin, sesame (tahini), sunflower

Nightshades or Spices Derived from Nightshades

Ashwagandha, capsicums/peppers, chili pepper flakes, chili powder, curry, cayenne pepper, paprika, pepinos, peppers (bell, chipotle, hot, red, and sweet), and pimentos; cape gooseberries, eggplant, goji berries (wolfberries), tobacco

Herbs and Spices

Allspice, anise, annatto, basil leaf, bay leaf, black caraway, cardamom, celery seed, chamomile, Chinese five-spice powder, chervil, chives, cilantro, coriander, cinnamon, cloves, cumin, curry powder, dill, fennel seed, fennel leaf, fenugreek, garlic, ginger, garam masala, juniper, kaffir lime leaf, lavender, lemongrass, mace, marjoram leaf, mustard, nutmeg, onion powder, oregano leaf, parsley, pepper, peppermint, poppy, rosemary, saffron, sage, savory leaf, sea or Himalayan salt, spearmint, tarragon, thyme, truffles, turmeric, vanilla

Flavorings

Watch for added ingredients

Anchovies or anchovy paste, apple cider vinegar, balsamic vinegar, capers, carob powder, coconut aminos (a soy sauce substitute), coconut concentrate, coconut milk, coconut water vinegar, fish sauce, vegetable juice (in moderation), red wine vinegar, truffle oil (made with olive oil), white wine vinegar

Sugar Alcohols

Erythritol, mannitol, malitol, sorbitol, xylitol

Sweeteners

In moderation

Allulose, monk fruit (Luo Han Guo), stevia

Alcohol

Not recommended, but if drinking, in extreme moderation

All beer, liquor, wine, or any other form of alcoholic beverages are technically not permitted. Some choose to have alcohol in moderation, distilled liquors like vodka, tequila, gin, or whiskey are the best choices with sparkling water and lemon or lime

Beverages

Water (club, mineral, reverse osmosis, seltzer, soda, sparkling [without natural flavors, sweeteners, and additives], spring); almond milk (unsweetened), coconut milk, coffee, green juices (fresh, without fruit), hemp milk (unsweetened), teas (black, green, or herbal), yerba mate

Foods and Beverages Included in Moderation

Bitter melon, cassava, chayote, coconut, coconut water, okra, pumpkin, squashes (all), winter melon, zucchini

KETO - FOODS TO AVOID

Grains and Grain-Like Foods

Amaranth, barley, buckwheat, bulgur, corn, farro, millet, oats/oatmeal, quinoa, rice, wild rice, rye, sorghum, spelt, teff, wheat (all varieties, including einkorn and semolina)

Berries

Acai, blackberry, blueberry, cranberry, currant, elderberry, Goji, gooseberry, grapes (all varieties), lingonberry, mulberry, raspberry, strawberry.

Rosaceae-family Fruits

Apple, apricot, cherry, nectarine, peach, pear, plum, quince, rosehip

Melons

Cantaloupe, honeydew, horned melon, melon pear, Persian melon, watermelon, winter melon

Citrus-family Fruits

Clementine, grapefruit, kumquat, orange, pomelo, tangelo, tangerine, yuzu

Tropical Fruits

Acerola, banana, chayote, cherimoya, date, dragon fruit, durian, fig, guava, jackfruit, kiwi, loquat, lychee, mango, mangosteen, papaya, passion fruit, pawpaw, persimmon, pineapple, plantain, pomegranate, star fruit, tamarind; all dried fruits

Vegetables

All varieties of peas, plantain, potatoes, string beans, sweet potatoes, taro, yam

Legumes

Adzuki beans, black beans, black-eyed peas, butter beans, calico beans, cannellini beans, chickpeas (garbanzo beans), fava beans (broad beans), great northern beans, green beans, Italian beans, kidney beans, lentils, lima beans, mung beans, navy beans, peanuts, peas, pinto beans, runner beans, soybeans (including edamame, tofu, tempeh, other soy products, and soy isolates, such as soy lecithin), split peas

Dairy

Ice cream, sweetened whipped cream, high-sugar yogurts

Processed Food Chemicals and Ingredients

Acrylamides, any ingredient with an unrecognizable chemical name, artificial and natural flavors, artificial food color, autolyzed protein, brominated vegetable oil, emulsifiers (carrageenan, cellulose gum, guar gum, lecithin, xanthan gum), hydrolyzed vegetable protein, monosodium glutamate, nitrates or nitrites (naturally occurring are okay), olestra, phosphoric acid, propylene glycol, textured vegetable protein, trans fats (partially hydrogenated vegetable oil, hydrogenated oil), yeast extract

Sugars

Agave, agave nectar, barley malt, barley malt syrup, beet sugar, brown rice syrup, brown sugar, cane crystals, cane juice, cane sugar, raw cane sugar, evaporated cane juice, and dehydrated cane juice, caramel, coconut sugar, coconut syrup, corn sweetener, corn syrup, and corn syrup solids, crystalline fructose, date sugar, demerara sugar, dextrin, dextrose, fructose, high-fructose corn syrup, fruit juice, fruit juice concentrate, glucose, glucose solids, golden syrup, honey, inulin, invert sugar, jaggery, lucuma, malt syrup, maltodextrin, maltose, maple syrup, molasses, muscovado sugar, palm sugar, raw sugar, refined sugar, rice bran syrup, rice syrup, saccharose, sorghum syrup, sucanat, sucrose, syrup, treacle, turbinado sugar, and yacon syrup

Beverages

Fruit juices of all kinds, electrolyte drinks, sweetened energy drinks, kombucha, soda (diet or regular), sweetened sports drinks

Alcohol

Beer, liquor, wine, or any other form of alcoholic beverage

LIFE AFTER KETO

I have many clients who follow Keto and are surprised by how much they enjoy the food choices along with the health benefits. Everyone is different and Keto must suit your lifestyle, so assess what's right for you.

Whether you remain on Keto for two weeks or two years, you will want to get out of ketosis slowly. To avoid weight gain, brain fog, sugar spikes, fatigue, bloating, and stomach upset, I highly recommend not adding more than one carbohydrate at a time and waiting another two to three days before introducing another carb. If you take it slowly and something upsets your stomach, you will be able to pinpoint which food caused the problem. Be patient and give it two to three weeks before adding carbs.

By this time the sugar cravings have been eliminated, I caution you to reintroduce sugar in your diet, should you be thinking of doing so, as it really takes one instance of sugar consumption for the system to ignite a craving. We don't need sugar, so I invite you to go as long as possible without it. You know how hard it is to dig out of that deep sugar hole!

In addition, I recommend that anyone getting off Keto to try and follow the Paleo FoodFrame, as this will continue to give you all the health benefits while giving you more variety of foods to eat in a less-restrictive eating plan.

KETO - RECIPES

Coco Avo Shake

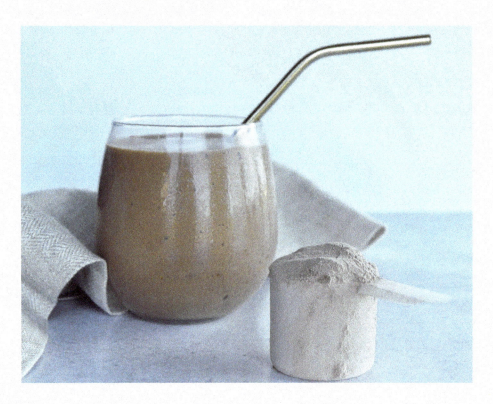

Ingredients:

1 cup coconut milk
1 scoop RGN Collagen Protein, chocolate
2 handfuls organic greens

½ avocado
1 cup ice

Instructions:

1. Blend all ingredients together until smooth.
2. Garnish with unsweetened shredded coconut or cacao nibs

Serves 1

Mini Quiche

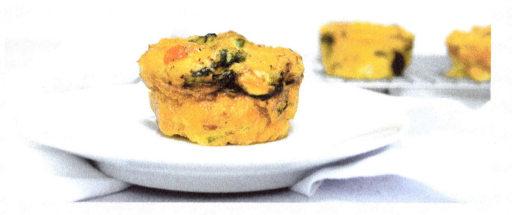

🍴 Ingredients:

6 eggs
¼ cup cherry tomatoes, diced
¼ yellow or white onion, diced
3 chicken sausages, cut in small pieces

½ cup spinach
1 ½ teaspoon coconut oil
Olive oil spray
Sea salt and pepper to taste

🍴 Instructions:

Preheat oven to 400 degrees.
Using a regular-sized muffin pan, grease muffin cups with olive oil spray.

1. Heat coconut oil on medium-low. Add tomatoes, onions, spinach, and sausages. Stirring frequently, cook for about 5 minutes or until spinach is limp and onions are translucent.
2. In a separate bowl, whisk together eggs, salt, and a little pepper. Add contents of veggies and sausages to eggs and fill muffin cups ¾ full and sprinkle a little black pepper.
3. Bake for 10-15 minutes or until the center is firm.
4. Cool in the pan one to two minutes before removing them from the tin.

Optional: Can use bacon instead of sausages. Can change up veggies and add herbs.

Makes 7 mini quiches

Avocado Spinach Dip

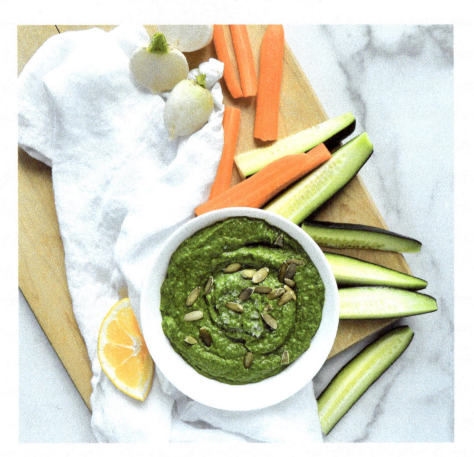

🍴 Ingredients:

1 ripe avocado
5 cups organic spinach
½ small white organic onion

2 garlic cloves
½ teaspoon sea salt
Juice of 1 lemon

🍴 Instructions:

Place all ingredients in a food processor and blend until well combined.

Serves 6-10

Olive Tapenade

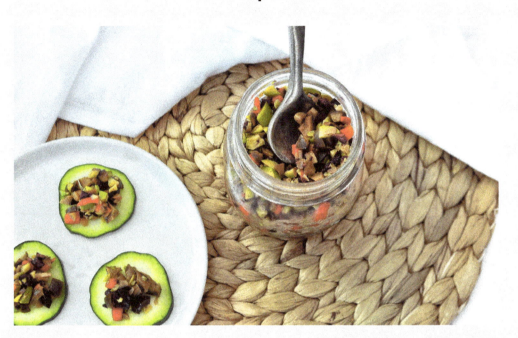

🍴 Ingredients:

2 garlic cloves, minced
¼ cup black olives, pitted
¼ cup Kalamata olives, pitted
¼ cup green olives, pitted

¼ cup roasted red peppers (optional)
Fresh black pepper to taste
2 long organic hot house cucumbers
Fennel greens for garnish

🍴 Instructions:

1. Combine garlic, olives and peppers in a food processor and process just enough to chop finely or chop everything by hand. Place in a bowl and add black pepper to taste. Refrigerate for about an hour.
2. Cut cucumbers into ¼-½" thick rounds. Place olive tapenade mixture on top and garnish with fennel fronds.

Serve immediately.

Serves 4-6

Crab Bisque

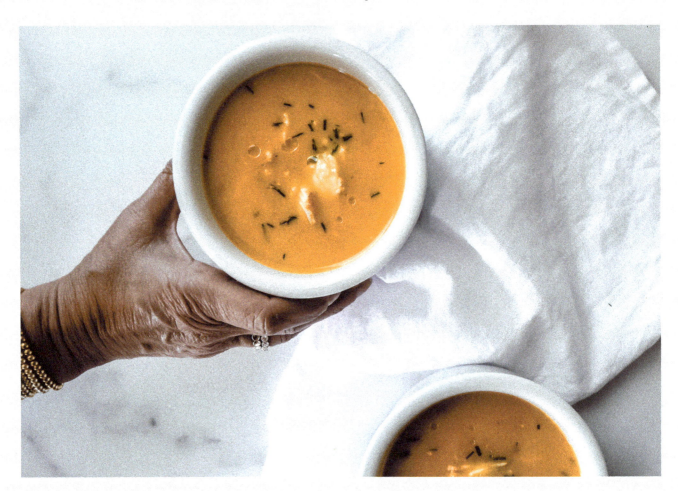

🍴 Ingredients:

2 tablespoons avocado oil
2 garlic cloves, chopped
1 yellow onion, chopped
1 pound of organic orange carrots, chopped
4 cups chicken bone broth
1 can (13.5 oz) full-fat coconut milk

1 pound crab meat (not imitation crab) cooked
1 tablespoon lemon juice
2 tablespoons fresh chives, cut into small (¼") segments
Sea salt and pepper to taste

Instructions:

1. In a large pot heat avocado oil over medium-high heat and sauté carrots, onions, and garlic for 10 minutes until lightly browned.
2. Add bone broth and coconut milk. Bring to a boil and reduce heat to medium-low. Cover and simmer until carrots are soft, about 10 minutes.
3. Using an immersion blender (or carefully transferring to a blender in batches), blend the mixture until creamy.
4. Add crabmeat, lemon juice, sea salt, and pepper and return to the stove top until heated through.
5. Sprinkle with chives and serve.

Serves 6

Thai Shrimp

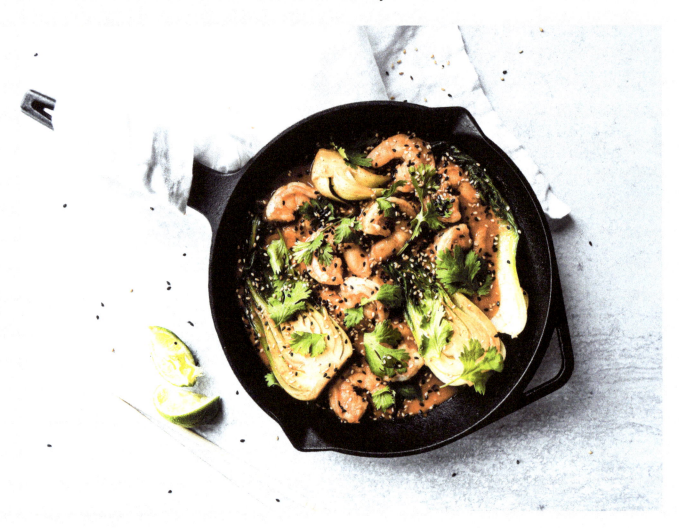

🍴 Ingredients:

1 pound of large raw shrimp, cleaned and trimmed (approximately 20-25)
1 tablespoon coconut oil
1 heaping tablespoon red chili paste
¼ cup full-fat coconut milk
1 cup cilantro, chopped

Instructions:

1. In a pan, melt coconut oil. Add shrimp and cook about 5-7 minutes until both sides are pink.
2. Add red chili paste and stir until shrimps are covered.
3. Add coconut milk and ½ cup cilantro. Cook for another 3 minutes. If you want it saucier, add more coconut milk.

Serve on a bed of cauliflower rice or quinoa and garnish with remaining cilantro.

Serves 4

Salmon Coconut Curry

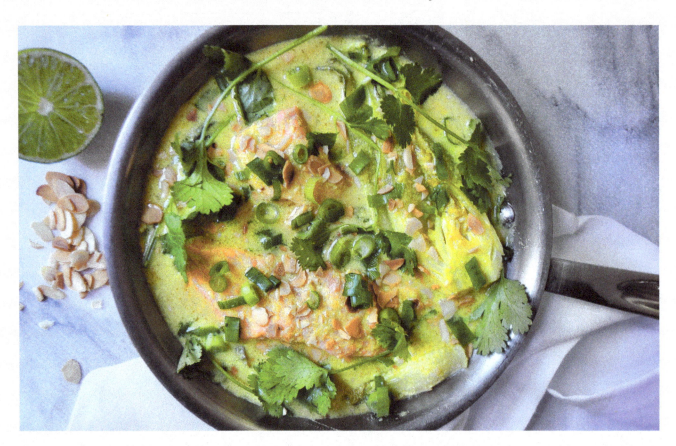

🍴 Ingredients:

4 salmon fillets
2 teaspoons sea salt
1 can full-fat coconut milk
¼ cup green curry paste
2 teaspoons minced ginger, skin removed
1 garlic clove, minced
1 head Bok choy (or 4 baby ones)

2 tablespoons fresh lime juice
4 scallions, thinly sliced
½ cup cilantro leaves
¼ cup roasted almond slivers
1 teaspoon ground turmeric
1 Serrano chili sliced into circles if wanting to add more spice (optional)

Instructions:

1. Season salmon with 1 teaspoon sea salt and let sit until ready to use.
2. In a large skillet, cook coconut milk, curry paste, ginger, garlic, and 1 teaspoon of sea salt over medium heat, stirring occasionally. Let simmer 5-6 minutes.
3. Cut Bok choy stems into ½-inch thick pieces and the leaves into 2-inch pieces. If using baby Bok choy, rinse, dry, and keep them whole. Add to cooking mixture and stir well.
4. Add salmon fillets in an even layer in the pan. Cover and cook over medium-low heat until salmon is cooked through and skin is opaque, about 6-8 minutes.
5. Remove skillet from heat and pour lime juice over the salmon.
6. Top with scallions, cilantro, almonds, and chili.

Optional: Serve with cauliflower rice.

Serves 4

Fudgy Collagen Brownies

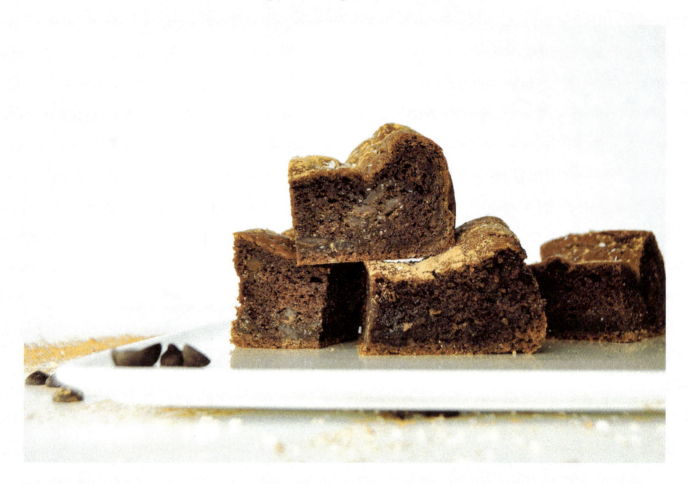

🍴 Ingredients:

4 eggs
½ cup monk fruit granules or coconut sugar
½ cup monk fruit flavored with maple syrup or regular maple syrup
2 tablespoons unsweetened almond or coconut milk
2 cups organic unsweetened almond butter or any nut butter

2 tablespoons blanched almond flour
4 scoops RGN Collagen Protein, chocolate
2 teaspoons baking soda
½ teaspoon sea salt
1-2 cups chocolate chips sweetened with monk fruit

Instructions:

Preheat oven to 350 degrees.

1. Combine wet and dry ingredients in separate bowls (without the chocolate chips).
2. Incorporate dry with wet ingredients. Mix in the chocolate chips.
3. Pour into an 8x8 cake pan lined with parchment paper for thicker brownies, or a 9x9 cake pan for thinner brownies.
4. Bake for 20 minutes. Be careful not to over-bake the brownies.

Makes 9 thick brownies

CHAPTER 6

THE AUTOIMMUNE PROTOCOL FOODFRAME

There are over 100 types of autoimmune diseases affecting over 50 million Americans. That's an astonishing 20 percent of the population!

While the exact number of people living with autoimmune disease is still unknown--because vast amounts of sufferers have not been diagnosed—the prevalence of these conditions is steadily increasing. Fortunately, you can do something about it. Diet and lifestyle affect the body with both cardiovascular disease and autoimmune disease. Type 2 diabetes, and obesity can trigger autoimmune conditions—but so can diet and lifestyle. You will often see vast improvements in symptoms by changing how you eat and changing behaviors like adding stress reduction practices, regular exercise, and good quality sleep. The Autoimmune Protocol (AIP) serves to support your immune system as well as your gut mucosa, the largest and most dynamic immunological environment in your body, by decreasing the foods that commonly cause inflammation.

ABOUT AUTOIMMUNE CONDITIONS

When your body perceives that it is under attack—whether from a virus, bacteria, parasite, or proteins —it creates antibodies that bind to specific proteins in these foreign cells to destroy them. Autoimmune disorders develop when your immune system mistakenly attacks your own tissues or glands. Normally, your immune system can distinguish between foreign cells and your own cells. When it doesn't, it releases proteins called autoantibodies that attack healthy cells. Some autoimmune diseases target only one organ while other diseases affect the entire body such as joints or skin.

In addition, we have Regulatory T Cells--protective cells that regulate inflammation and that are commonly referred to as T Reg Cells. These are white blood cells that develop in the thymus gland; when matured, they will regulate or dysregulate the immune system. When an autoimmune disease is present, the TH17 T reg-cells become activated and can trigger a cascade of systemic inflammation.

There are three phases of autoimmunity:

1. **Silent autoimmunity.** This is when the onset of immune self-tolerance takes place. The antibodies are present but without symptoms or signs as tissue has not yet been damaged.
2. **Autoimmune reactivity.** In this stage, the tissue or organ destruction becomes noticeable due to loss of function. It might not yet be diagnosed as an autoimmune disease.
3. **Autoimmune disease.** This phase is when a person is typically diagnosed as a result of positive testing via blood tests, imaging, or nerve conduction (a medical diagnostic test to determine nerve damage).

Common Autoimmune Diseases

Addison's Disease
Alopecia Areata
Celiac Disease
Crohn's Disease
Diabetes – Type 1
Endometriosis
Eczema
Fibromyalgia
Grave's Disease
Hashimoto's Thyroiditis
Lupus
Meniere's Syndrome
Multiple Sclerosis
PANDAS (Pediatric Autoimmune Neuropsychiatric Disorders Associated with Streptococcal Infections)
Primary Biliary Cirrhosis
Psoriasis
Raynaud's Syndrome
Restless Leg Syndrome
Rheumatoid Arthritis
Sjogren's Syndrome
Ulcerative Colitis

Symptoms of Common Autoimmune Diseases

Symptoms tend to be vague and accumulate slowly, which makes an autoimmune condition challenging to catch before it escalates. The average patient with an autoimmune disease will see an average of *six doctors* before being diagnosed—and, on average, it takes *4.6 years* to get an accurate diagnosis! One of the reasons for this is that there is currently no medical specialty devoted to the diagnosis and treatment of autoimmune disease, just symptom management.

Common symptoms can range from the annoying to debilitating, and include:

- Allergies
- Anxiety
- Attention deficit issues
- Body rashes; acne, dermatitis, eczema, psoriasis, red bumps, red flaking skin, rosacea
- Brain fog
- Cold extremities
- Constipation

- Digestive issues; bloating, constipation, cramping, diarrhea, gas
    - Dry mouth and eyes
    - Frequent colds and coughs
    - Fatigue or hyperactivity
    - Headaches and migraines
    - Muscle stiffness, pain, and weakness
    - Thinning hair
    - Weight gain or loss

Contributing Factors to Autoimmune Diseases

Research is still uncovering the specific causes and treatments of autoimmune conditions, but we do know that they are the perfect storm of factors resulting in the body's inability to recognize a normal cell from invader cells. The attacks will continue until the process is disrupted, which is why the condition can exist for a long time before symptoms become present and are able to eventually be diagnosed. If left untreated, the body begins to break down or destroy the gland or tissue that it perceives as the enemy.

Because my own autoimmune condition was undiagnosed for so long, and I have extensively studied these issues. I learned that there is no one root cause or definable trigger—unlike certain other diseases that are wholly genetic or caused by a specific situation; a person with a rare cancer called mesothelioma, for example, has almost always developed it after exposure to asbestos over time. Sometimes there is just one major factor, but usually there is a perfect storm of several factors. In addition, I test every client for thyroid antibodies unless they are showing other symptoms like arthritis; if so, I will test for those antibodies. In the stool test I order, there is an entire section that shows potential autoimmune triggers. For example, I have yet to have a client with rheumatoid arthritis who does not have the bacteria Prevotella Species. Certain parasites can trigger autoimmunity as well.

In other words, most people have a combination of root causes and/or genetic predisposition. I always test each new clients' autoimmunity, as so many people have one or more of these contributing factors:

Immutable Conditions

- Gender - Approximately 75 % of autoimmune sufferers are women
- Having one autoimmune disease increases the likelihood of being diagnosed with more

Root Causes, in descending order of likelihood

- Genetics - Roughly one-third of autoimmune conditions are genetic. A specific gene called HLA-B27 is associated with some autoimmune diseases
- Leaky gut – Also known as intestinal permeability. This is a major contributor to autoimmune disease
- Bacteria/Parasite - Certain bacteria and parasites found in the gut through comprehensive stool

testing are known to be potential autoimmune triggers
- Infections That Are Persistent – Can be dormant infections that are viral, such as Epstein Barr or cytomegalovirus; bacterial, fungal, or parasitical
- Heavy Metals – Storing excessive amounts in the body, unable to detoxify them
- Toxins – A high toxin overload
- MTHFR – A gene mutation (see p.40 in Chapter 2)
- Vitamin Deficiency – Especially vitamin D
- Nutrient-poor Diet and Food Sensitivities - Mostly to dairy, gluten, grains, and soy
- Lifestyle – Chronic stress, lack of exercise, highly processed food diet, insufficient sleep

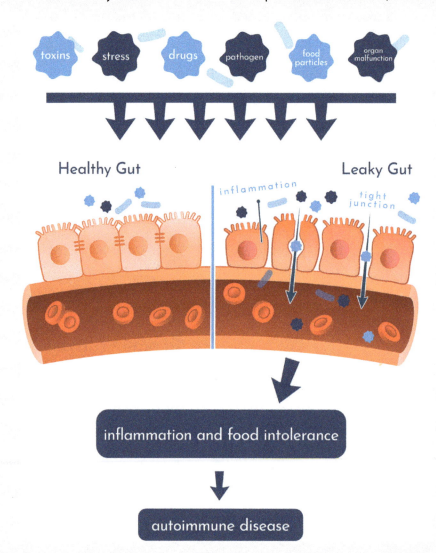

Leaky Gut Syndrome

Among the biggest pieces of the pie that cause autoimmune disease are genetics, which you can't control; toxins, which you read about in Chapter 3; and leaky gut.

Intestinal permeability is the clinical term for leaky gut, which basically means there are holes or fissures in the intestinal lining. [Illustration leaky gut] There is only one layer of skin on your mucosal lining to protect it. Villi, small hair-like particles, live on top of that skin and absorb vitamins and minerals--but if destroyed, they do not regrow unless gluten is fully removed from the diet.

In addition, gluten, sugar, alcohol, and processed foods are effective villi-destroyers—and fewer villi means that openings in the intestinal lining, called tight junctions, can develop. Undigested proteins, pathogens, toxins, and bacteria can now leak through the microscopic holes in your intestinal lining and enter directly into your bloodstream or lymphatic system. Your body sees them as invaders and begins to produce antibodies to attack and destroy them. This attack can take place all day and night and is directly responsible for triggering the T Reg cells to create an inflammation storm. Therefore, when your body has an autoimmune disease, it is in a constant state of inflammation. Remember, 75-85 percent of your immune system is produced in the gut, so this has a significant impact on your immune system.

This is why diet is so critical to health! Bear in mind, too, that just because your family has autoimmunity doesn't mean you can't prevent leaky gut if you act early and before there are any symptoms. But if your leaky gut is never fixed, disease and inflammation will proliferate. Cells in the intestinal wall regenerate every 72 hours as long as they are not being exposed to gluten, so when ordering a stool test for a client, if I suspect there is leaky gut, I will add zonulin to the order. Zonulin is a protein that is secreted into the gut if leaky gut exists. That way leaky gut can be definitively identified, and you will have a quantitative number to work with.

More About Gluten

Another contributing factor to autoimmune disease is gluten.

I know what you're thinking—is gluten really that bad? Isn't it just a fad? I eat gluten and feel fine! Well, sometimes it's fine, but when it's not, you can really suffer. Gluten is an inflammatory food and if you are not celiac, you will most likely not have a physical reaction when eating it--but you will have a silent inflammatory response. The stool test I use looks for Anti-Gliadin (the protein in gluten) IgA, the antibody to gluten which will determine the degree of sensitivity you have to it.

Gluten is not a protein itself but rather a protein composite, which means it's composed of several different proteins. It's found in grass-like grains, such as wheat, barley, rye, kamut, and spelt. The flour milled from those grains is used primarily in bread, pasta, cereals, and baked goods. It provides an elasticity and glue-like capacity to hold these grains together and provide them with a chewy texture.

The primary proteins giving gluten its utility in baking and its difficulty in health are glutenin and gliadin (in wheat), secalin (in rye), and hordein (in barley). These are elastic proteins in the protein family known as prolamins. This unique protein composite is insoluble in water and comes from the endosperm within the seeds of grass-related grains. Our current version of gluten is more scientifically engineered than in previous generations, with the intent of producing doughier and fluffier pastries along with a more water-soluble form to be used in things like shampoo and lunch meat. This leaves us more exposed to gluten now than ever before. In addition, our bodies do not have the digestive enzymes necessary to break down these new types of prolamins, and this can contribute to gut dysbiosis, an imbalance of good and bad gut bacteria.

Gluten affects autoimmune conditions in several ways. It is known to cause leaky gut; stimulate the production of zonulin; contribute to gut imbalances like Candida (a type of yeast) overgrowth and SIBO (Small Intestinal Bacteria Overgrowth); spark the production of antibodies that cause attacks to your tissues, organs, or glands; and trigger inflammation.

Gluten Intolerance

Gluten intolerance is separated into three distinct categories: Celiac Disease, Non-Celiac Gluten Sensitivity, and Wheat Allergy.

*Celiac Disease is estimated to affect one percent of the population and has the same root causes as the other diseases listed in this section. It is usually diagnosed via antibodies from blood tests as well as intestinal biopsies. It develops when the proteins in gluten (primarily gliadin but also glutenin) trigger your immune system to overreact with strong and unusual antibodies. As this autoimmune response slowly flattens the villi, you become less and less able to process any nutrition from your food. Celiac disease also triggers inflammation of the intestinal wall. The combination of absorption-killing villous atrophy and inflammation sets off a domino-effect of increasingly serious health problems.

*Non-Celiac Gluten Sensitivity, on the other hand, is not hereditary, but is far more common, although it is a little more difficult to pinpoint. Researchers estimate 18 million Americans have gluten sensitivity; their symptoms are similar to those with Celiac Disease, but the blood test and biopsy used to identify and diagnose Celiac Disease is negative, as is a test for a wheat allergy. The only way to confidently diagnose Non-Celiac Gluten Sensitivity is through deduction (after a patient tests negative for Celiac Disease and a wheat allergy) and through a gluten challenge, where this pesky protein composite is removed from the diet for a period, then slowly re-introduced while changes in health and symptoms are observed.

*Wheat allergy triggers are fundamentally different from Celiac Disease symptoms, but they are often inaccurately referred to as gluten allergy symptoms. A wheat allergy is a histamine response to wheat, much like a peanut allergy or hay fever. Wheat allergies manifest themselves in many ways, which can be quite different for different people. Some people experience hives while others might experience stomach pain. A wheat allergy, unlike Celiac Disease, is considered a Type 1 Hypersensitivity, which is an allergic reaction caused by an exposure to a specific allergen. It is important to make this distinction: Celiac Disease is not a Type 1 Hypersensitivity, and most Celiac patients consuming gluten experience immediate pain or discomfort—but, rarely, others do not. Someone with a wheat allergy, however, will experience problems soon after they eat wheat.

Recent research and current gluten intolerance statistics suggest that 10-15 % of the population may suffer from some form of intolerance, yet a vast majority of these individuals have not yet been accurately diagnosed. Furthermore, we now know even patients who test negative for Celiac Disease may suffer from some form of undiagnosed non-Celiac gluten intolerance.

Symptoms of Gluten Sensitivity

There are over 250 documented symptoms of a gluten sensitivity, and their manifestation varies greatly from person to person. Here are both the most common and important symptoms you should know about on the gluten intolerance checklist:

- Abdominal bloating, pain, or cramping; alternating bouts of diarrhea and constipation; malodorous flatulence and stools; grayish stools; stomach rumbling
- Anemia
- Back pain
- Bone density loss
- Canker sores or mouth ulcers
- Depression, anxiety, and irritability
- Dry Hair
- Dermatitis Herpetiformis
- Fatigue
- Gluten Ataxia
- Headaches and migraines
- Joint pain
- Nausea
- Peripheral Neuropathy (including either a tingling or sensation of swelling in toes and fingers)
- Stunted growth and failure to thrive
- Vitamin and mineral deficiencies
- Vomiting
- Unexplained weight loss

One key point to consider is that gluten is in more foods and products than you may realize. If you think removing gluten from your diet involves just avoiding bread and baked goods, I'm afraid you're mistaken. It is often used in sauces, flavorings, flavor enhancers, and even as a binder or filler in medications, vitamins, and supplements.

Adapting a true gluten-free diet requires more than just removing wheat products from your lifestyle. Because it is not just a sensitivity for those with autoimmune issues--you need to become diligent, especially in restaurants, as only a tiny bit of gluten can potentially have lasting inflammatory effects. Studies show that an inflammatory response from a little bit of gluten can last up to six months.

HOW THE AIP (AUTOIMMUNE PROTOCOL) WORKS

AIP is intended to be an elimination diet lasting 30-90 days. This protocol is close to the Paleo lifestyle but with a few more restrictions. In addition to what Paleo removes, AIP also removes nuts, seeds, eggs, and nightshades due to their allergy potential and possible inflammatory response.

I recommend adhering to this eating plan for 90 days, then slowly reintroduce foods one at a time to see if there is a reaction. If any kind of reaction occurs, remove that food and try again in another 90 days or more. If a reaction persists with those foods, consider removing them indefinitely. Your body will communicate with you so train yourself to listen.

WHAT THE AIP IS BEST FOR

Take heart because the autoimmune protocol is recommended for anyone who has an autoimmune disease. Even if you're in perfect health and have not been diagnosed with an autoimmune disease, you can still follow this diet and reap its benefits. It is perfect for the person who has one or two parents and/or siblings with an autoimmune disease and would like to increase their odds in preventing it in their future. This is where genetics can increase the likelihood of developing this condition but doesn't mean you don't have a fighting chance to prevent it. Being proactive can be life-changing for those with the genes.

The AIP supports the healing process of the immune system and gut mucosa, the largest and most dynamic immunological environment of the body. It accomplishes this by decreasing inflammatory foods which perpetuate the immune response. Another benefit of the AIP is that it helps identify foods that trigger symptoms, so it can prevent flare-ups.

The very first study of the AIP eating lifestyle and autoimmune status was conducted at the Scripps Clinic in La Jolla, California and reported in 2017. The researchers and physicians tracked 15 autoimmune sufferers who had either Ulcerative Colitis or Crohn's disease. They followed a strict AIP and within six weeks, clinical remission was achieved by 11 of the 15 participants.

The AIP is perfect to go on anytime, especially if you are having flare-ups. Also, if you or an immediate blood relative has an autoimmune disease, I highly recommend you eliminate gluten from your diet completely.

There is no limit to how many times you can do this protocol, so you might want to revisit it at least once or twice a year. It will make you feel so much better, so take advantage of it when you need it. And even though it is meant to be followed for 30-90 days, if it works for you, stay on it for as long as you like. Although it is restrictive, it can only do a body good.

SIDEBAR – Kerri's Story

Kerri walked in my office and said it was her last stop. This vibrant 69-year-old woman had recently retired and had a long list of destinations and excursions that she and her husband had planned. She was thin and terribly ill, having been diagnosed with Microscopic Colitis, an intestinal ailment six months ago and had gone down the mainstream medical rabbit hole. Multiple doctors offered her many different medications, but nothing worked. Nearly every day, Kerri experienced chronic diarrhea starting in the middle of the night, which woke her several times, and then continued until late morning just about daily. She could not plan any appointments before noon and would occasionally experience urgent diarrhea if she ate something that her body did not like. In addition, she had chronic urinary tract infections.

Kerri decided to seek alternative options and was willing to change her diet. After ordering blood work and a stool test, I found the culprit. Kerri had Campylobacter and Citrobacter freundii, both pathogenic root causes of colitis. She also had significant inflammation in her intestines. I put Kerri on the Autoimmune Protocol and she started getting better in about two weeks. All her diarrhea disappeared entirely by week three. I also chose food and supplements to help decrease the inflammation to support the healing of her gut.

We retested her stool after eight weeks and it had improved immensely, but the infections were not entirely gone. After another round of natural anti-bacterial and anti-microbial supplements, she finally received the all-clear. Kerri has stayed on the AIP protocol and feels amazing. Every time she pops into my office for more collagen protein, she has either just returned or preparing to leave on a fabulous trip.

WHO SHOULD AVOID THE AIP

This diet is aimed at decreasing inflammation, so anyone can benefit from it at any age. There really isn't anyone that can't follow it. I recommend the AIP for anyone who has been diagnosed with, has immediate family with, or who suspects they have an autoimmune condition but does not have a conclusive diagnosis.

AIP FOODS TO ENJOY

Meat *Includes broth and collagen*

Cattle (beef, veal), deer (venison), goat, hare, pig (pork), rabbit, sheep (lamb, mutton), wild game (buffalo/bison, boar, elk)

Poultry

Chicken, duck, goose, grouse, guinea hen, ostrich, pheasant, quail, turkey

Fish

Anchovy, arctic char, bass, bonito, carp, catfish, cod, eel, gar, haddock, hake, halibut, herring, mackerel, mahi-mahi, marlin, monkfish, perch, pollock, salmon, sardine, snapper, sole, swordfish, tilapia, trout, tuna (ahi, yellowfin), turbot, walleye

Shellfish

Clams, crab, crawfish, lobster, mussels, octopus, oysters, scallops, shrimp, squid

Dairy

Ghee, milks, and yogurts made with coconut milk

Leafy Vegetables

Arugula, beet greens, Bok choy, broccoli rabe, Brussels sprouts, cabbage, carrot tops, celery, chicory, collard greens, cress, dandelion greens, endive, kale (all varieties), lettuce (all varieties), mustard greens, Napa cabbage, purslane, radicchio, sorrel, spinach, swiss chard, tatsoi, turnip greens, watercress

Non-starchy Vegetables

Artichoke, asparagus, broccoli, cauliflower, celery, fennel, rhubarb (stems only), squash blossoms.

Allium-family Vegetables

Chive, garlic, leek, onion, scallion, shallot, wild leek

Roots, Tubers, and Bulb Vegetables

Arrowroot, bamboo shoot, beet, burdock, carrot, cassava, celeriac, daikon, ginger, horseradish, Jerusalem artichoke, jicama, kohlrabi, lotus root, parsnip, radish, rutabaga, sweet potato, taro, turnip, wasabi, water chestnut, yam

Sea Vegetables

Arame, dulse, hijiki, kombu, nori, wakame

Vegetable-like Fruits

Avocado, bitter melon, chayote, cucumber, okra, olives, plantain, pumpkin, squash, winter melon, zucchini

Berries

Acai, blackberry, blueberry, cranberry, currant, elderberry, gooseberry, grapes (all varieties), lingonberry, mulberry, raspberry, strawberry

Rosaceae-family Fruits

Apple, apricot, cherry, nectarine, peach, pear, plum, quince, rosehip

Melons

Cantaloupe, honeydew, horned melon, melon pear, Persian melon, watermelon, winter melon

Citrus-family Fruits

Clementine, grapefruit, kumquat, lemon, lime, orange, pomelo, tangelo, tangerine, yuzu

Tropical Fruits

Acerola, banana, chayote, cherimoya, coconut, date, dragon fruit, durian, fig, guava, jackfruit, kiwi, loquat, lychee, mango, mangosteen, papaya, passion fruit, pawpaw, persimmon, pineapple, plantain, pomegranate, star fruit, tamarind

Edible Fungi/Mushrooms

Chanterelle, Cremini, morel, oyster, porcini, Portobello, shiitake, truffle

Animal Fats

Bacon fat, lard, leaf lard (fat from pig), pan drippings, poultry fat, schmaltz (chicken or goose fat), strutto (clarified pork fat), tallow (from beef, lamb, or mutton)

Plant Fats

Avocado oil (cold-pressed), coconut oil, olive oil (cold-pressed), palm oil, palm shortening, and red palm oil

Probiotic Foods

Fermented meat or fish, kombucha, kvass, lacto-fermented fruits and vegetables, non-dairy kefir, sauerkraut

Herbs and Spices

Basil leaf, bay leaf, cardamom, chamomile, chervil, chives, cilantro, coriander, cinnamon, cloves, curry leaf, dill, fennel, garlic, ginger, kaffir lime leaf, lavender, lemongrass, mace, marjoram leaf, onion powder, oregano leaf, parsley, black pepper, peppermint, rosemary, saffron, sage, savory leaf, sea or Himalayan salt, spearmint, tarragon, thyme, truffles, turmeric, vanilla

Flavorings

Watch for added ingredients

Anchovies or anchovy paste, apple cider vinegar, balsamic vinegar, capers, carob powder, coconut aminos (soy sauce substitute), coconut concentrate, coconut milk, coconut water vinegar, fish sauce, fruit and vegetable juices (in moderation), organic jams and chutneys, red wine vinegar, truffle oil (made with olive oil), vanilla, white wine vinegar

Sweeteners

In moderation

Coconut sugar, coconut syrup, honey, maple sugar, maple syrup, molasses, trace amounts of cane sugar are okay in cured meats

Foods and Beverages Included in Moderation

Coconut, fruit juices (less than 10–20 grams per day), green or black tea, kombucha, moderate to high glycemic load fruits/vegetables (dried fruit, plantain, taro, etc.), omega-6 polyunsaturated fat-rich foods (poultry and industrially raised fatty meat), yerba mate

AIP FOODS TO AVOID

Grains and Grain-Like Foods

Amaranth, barley, buckwheat, bulgur, corn, farro, millet, oats/oatmeal, quinoa, any type of rice, rye, sorghum, spelt, teff, wheat (all varieties, including einkorn and semolina)

Dairy

Butter, buttermilk, cheese (all types), cream (all varieties), dairy-protein isolates, ice cream, kefir, milk, curds, whey, whey-protein isolate, yogurt

Eggs

Chicken, duck, goose, quail, including fish eggs/caviar

Legumes

Adzuki beans, black beans, black-eyed peas, butter beans, calico beans, cannellini beans, chickpeas (garbanzo beans), fava beans (broad beans), great northern beans, green beans, Italian beans, kidney beans, lentils, lima beans, mung beans, navy beans, peanuts, peas, pinto beans, runner beans, soybeans (including edamame, tofu, tempeh, other soy products, and soy isolates, such as soy lecithin), split peas

Processed Vegetable Oils

Canola oil (rapeseed oil), corn oil, cottonseed oil, grapeseed oil, palm kernel oil, peanut oil, safflower oil, soybean oil, sunflower oil

Processed Food Chemicals and Ingredients

Acrylamides, any ingredient with an unrecognized chemical name, artificial and natural flavors, artificial food color, autolyzed protein, brominated vegetable oil, emulsifiers (carrageenan, cellulose gum, guar gum, lecithin, xanthan gum), hydrolyzed vegetable protein, monosodium glutamate, nitrates or nitrites (naturally occurring are okay), olestra, phosphoric acid, propylene glycol, textured vegetable protein, trans fats (partially hydrogenated vegetable oil, hydrogenated oil), yeast extract

Sugars

Agave, agave nectar, barley malt, barley malt syrup, beet sugar, brown rice syrup, brown sugar, cane crystals, cane juice, cane sugar, raw cane sugar, evaporated cane juice, dehydrated cane juice, caramel, corn sweetener, corn syrup, and corn syrup solids, crystalline fructose, date sugar, demerara sugar, dextrin, dextrose, fructose, high-fructose corn syrup, fruit juice, fruit juice concentrate, glucose, glucose solids, golden syrup, inulin, invert sugar, jaggery, lactose, malt syrup, maltodextrin, maltose, monk fruit (Luo Han Guo), muscovado sugar, palm sugar, raw sugar, refined sugar, rice bran syrup, rice syrup, saccharose, sorghum syrup, sucanat, sucrose, syrup, treacle, turbinado sugar, and yacon syrup

Sugar Alcohols

Naturally occurring sugar alcohols found in whole foods like fruit are okay

Erythritol, mannitol, sorbitol, xylitol

Non-nutritive Sweeteners

Acesulfame potassium, aspartame, neotame, saccharin (Sweet n' Low, Equal), stevia, sucralose (Splenda)

Nuts and Nut Oils

Coconut is okay because it's not a nut

Any flavors, flours, butters, oils, whole nuts, or other products derived from: Almonds, Brazil nuts, cashews, chestnuts, hazelnuts, macadamia, pecans, pine nuts, pistachios, walnuts

Seeds and Seed Oils

Any flavors, butters, oils, and other products derived from; Chia, chocolate (dark or milk), cocoa, coffee, flax, hemp seeds, poppy seeds, pumpkin seeds, sesame seeds, sunflower seeds

Nightshades or Spices Derived from Nightshades

Ashwagandha, capsicums/peppers, chili pepper flakes, chili powder, curry, cayenne pepper, paprika, pepinos, peppers (bell, chipotle, hot, red, and sweet), and pimentos; cape gooseberries (ground cherries, not regular cherries), eggplant, goji berries (wolfberries), potatoes (sweet potatoes and yams are not nightshades and are okay), sweet plantains, tobacco, tomatoes (all varieties)

Spices

Allspice, anise, annatto, black caraway (Russian caraway, black cumin), cardamom, celery seed, coriander, cumin, dill seed, fennel seed, fenugreek, juniper, mustard, nutmeg, pepper, poppy

Spice Blends

Chinese five-spice powder (contains star anise, peppercorn, and fennel seed), curry powder (often contains coriander seed, cumin seed, and cardamom), garam masala (contains cumin), poultry seasoning (often contains peppercorn and nutmeg), steak seasoning (often contains peppercorn, chili pepper, cumin seed, cayenne pepper, fenugreek, and red pepper)

Alcohol

Small amounts in kombucha are okay

Beer, liquor, wine, or any other form of alcoholic beverage

Beverages

CBD and hemp drinks, coffee, energy drinks, flavored and functional water, sodas

LIFE AFTER THE AIP

Once you have brought back certain foods, I recommend that you try to maintain a looser AIP, which resembles more of a Paleo plan. Continue to refrain from eating any legumes, grains, nightshades, and dairy, but it's possible to have these foods very occasionally. In my experience, many people do not do well with nightshades, especially people with autoimmune disease. I would encourage you to do the best you can to remove them entirely or enjoy them on rare occasions. Then bring back nuts, seeds, and eggs. I also recommend that you avoid gluten (which falls into the grain category) altogether, as that has lasting inflammatory effects on autoimmune conditions for up to 90 days, or in some cases six months.

AIP - RECIPES

Chai Latte Shake

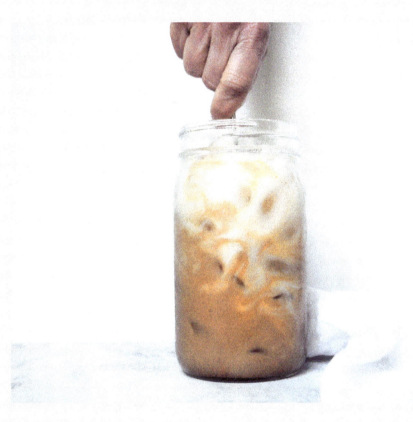

🍴 Ingredients:

1 scoop RGN Collagen Protein, vanilla
⅓ banana (fresh or frozen)
1 heaping teaspoon ground cinnamon
1 heaping teaspoon ground ginger

½ teaspoon ground cloves
½ teaspoon vanilla powder
½ cup ice

🍴 Instructions:

Blend all ingredients together until smooth. Can garnish with cinnamon.

Serves 1

Risa Groux, CN

Mashed Cauliflower

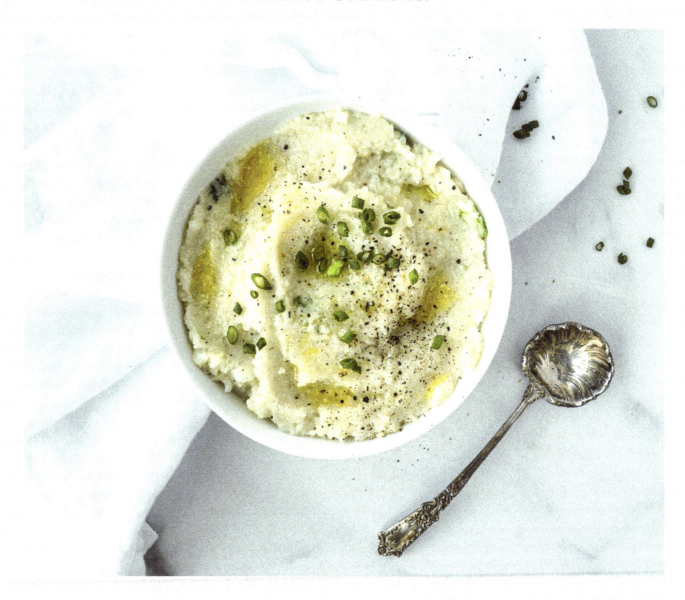

Ingredients:

1-1 ½ heads of raw organic cauliflower (thick stem removed)
2 cloves garlic
¼ cup full fat coconut milk
2-4 tablespoons fresh horseradish (depending how strong you like it)
1 tablespoon chives minced
Sea salt and pepper to taste

Instructions:

1. Steam cauliflower florets until soft (approximately 20 minutes). Strain or blot using a paper towel to remove excess water.
2. Place in a food processor with garlic and slowly add the coconut milk and horseradish. For a thicker consistency add less liquid.
3. Stir in chives, sea salt, and pepper.

Optional: For a richer taste, you can add ghee if desired.

Serves 4-6

Creamy Asparagus Soup

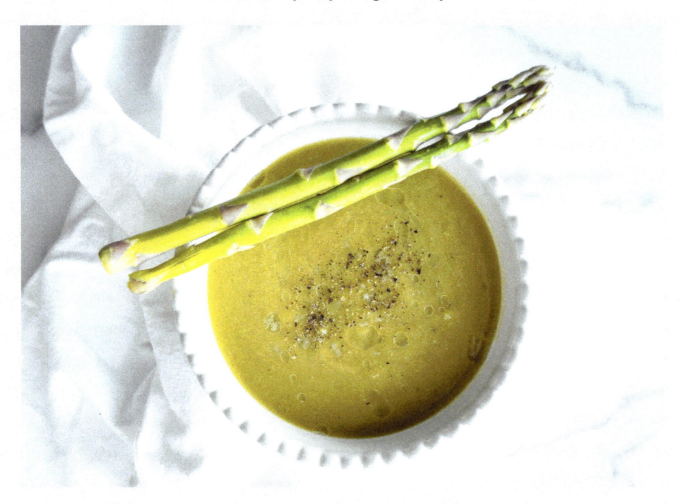

🍴 Ingredients:

½ head of organic cauliflower, cored and chopped
2-3 tablespoons coconut oil
1 medium onion, diced
4 garlic cloves, chopped

2 pounds of fresh asparagus (2-3 bunches) ends trimmed and cut onto 2-inch pieces. Reserve a few tips for garnish
4 cups of chicken or vegetable broth
1 large piece of lemon peel, approximately 2" x 1"
Sea salt and black pepper to taste

Instructions:

1. In a soup pan on medium heat, melt coconut oil and sauté garlic and onions until translucent, about 5-7 minutes.
2. Add chopped asparagus and sauté for 3-5 minutes while stirring.
3. Pour in the chicken or vegetable broth and add the lemon peel and cauliflower pieces.
4. Bring soup to a boil, then simmer for 15 minutes.
5. Remove lemon peel and use immersion blender to puree until smooth.
6. Add sea salt and black pepper to taste.
7. Cut asparagus tips in half, (length wise) and top the soup with them before serving.

Serves 4-6

Italian Turkey Meatballs

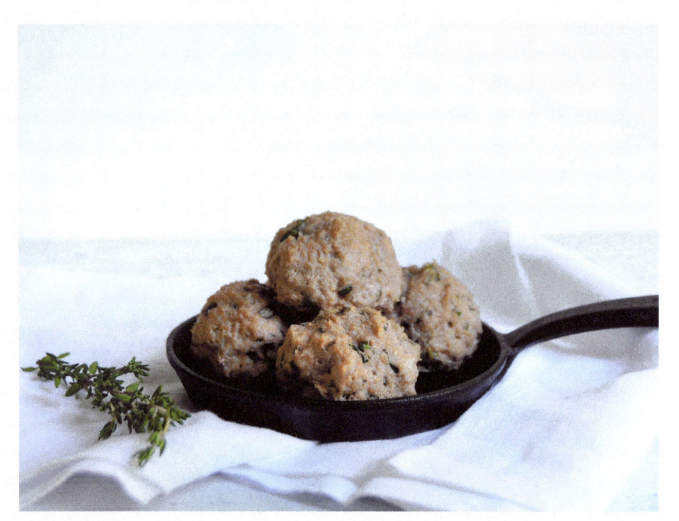

Ingredients:

1 lb. organic ground turkey
2 garlic cloves, minced
1 tablespoon fresh thyme
1 tablespoon fresh oregano

1 tablespoon fresh basil, chopped
1 teaspoon sea salt
½ teaspoon freshly ground black pepper

Instructions:

Preheat oven to 350 degrees.

1. In a bowl, add turkey, garlic, thyme, oregano, basil, salt, and pepper. Mix with your hands until well combined. With slightly wet hands, form meatballs that are approximately 1 ½-inches to 2-inches in diameter and place on a cookie sheet lined with parchment paper.
2. Cook for 20 minutes and serve.

Serve with mashed cauliflower or cauliflower rice.

Serves 4-6

Risa Groux, CN

Sweet Potato Fries

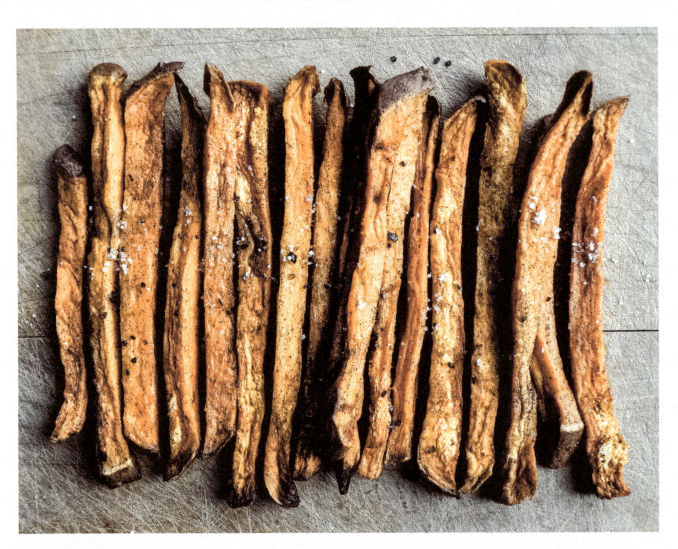

🍴 Ingredients:

2 sweet potatoes or yams, medium size
Olive oil, drizzle
¼ teaspoon sea salt
½ teaspoon cinnamon

Instructions:

Preheat oven to 400 degrees.

1. Wash and dry the sweet potatoes. Cut off the ends. Cut the potatoes vertically into fries, half an inch thick.
2. Transfer to a bowl and drizzle with olive oil to lightly coat the pieces. Sprinkle with sea salt and cinnamon. Mix well.
3. Place the fries on top of a metal cooling rack over a cookie sheet and place in the oven. Bake for 40-60 minutes, turning halfway through.
4. If you like crispy fries, broil for 2-4 minutes.

Serves 4-6

Cinnamon Cookies

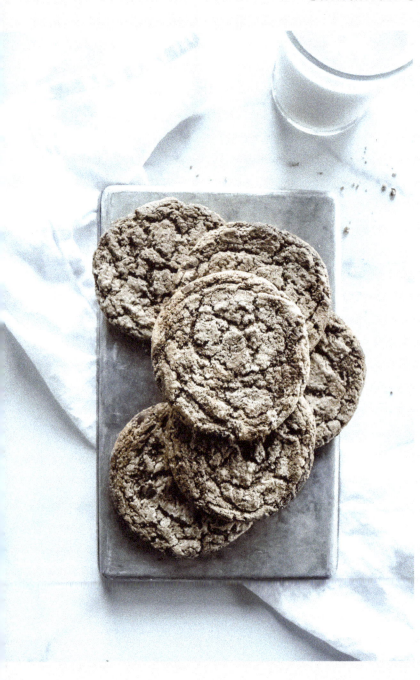

🍴 Ingredients:

1 cup tiger nut flour
¾ cup arrowroot flour
1 teaspoon baking soda
¼ teaspoon fine sea salt
1 teaspoon ground cinnamon
½ cup palm shortening
¼ cup maple syrup
1 scoop RGN Collagen Protein, vanilla
¼-½ cup carob chips

🍴 Instructions:

Preheat oven to 350 degrees.

1. In a large bowl, mix tiger nut flour, arrowroot flour, baking soda, sea salt, and cinnamon.
2. In a small pot, melt the shortening and add maple syrup. Mix well. Add collagen and continue to stir until there are no clumps.
3. Pour the liquid ingredients over the dry ones and stir until it becomes a dough.
4. With your hands, roll the batter into small balls and place on a parchment covered cookie sheet. Flatten the cookie balls slightly. If using carob chips, gently press them onto the cookies. Place in the oven and bake for 12 minutes.

Makes 10-12 cookies

CHAPTER 7

THE VEGAN FOODFRAME

The Vegan FoodFrame is plant-based and abstains from any animal foods or food products—that means no dairy, eggs, fish, seafood, poultry, or meat of any kind. Some people choose to be vegan for ethical, environmental, or religious reasons. It is undeniable that the environmental impact created by animal agriculture is harming our planet: 65 percent of the total nitrous oxide emissions; 35-40 percent of global methane emissions; and 9 percent of global carbon dioxide emissions come from animal agriculture (these are the greenhouse gasses involved in air pollution and climate change). Between 550-5,200 gallons of water are needed to produce a single pound of beef--43 times more water than is needed to produce a single pound of cereal grain!

Others prefer to eat nutrient-dense plant-based foods so they feel better, as there is evidence that eating a diet comprised of mostly plant foods, has numerous health benefits, mainly due to lower levels of saturated fat. Plant-based diets have been linked to the reduction of heart disease, cancer, Type 2 diabetes, and weight loss. Eliminating dairy products can reduce inflammation and blood sugar levels while decreasing dairy and meat will reduce the consumption of toxins, hormones, and antibiotics, as these are routinely given to dairy cows and cattle.

The difference between vegan and vegetarian diets:

- **Vegans:** Do not eat meat, poultry, fish, or any products derived from animals, including eggs, dairy products, honey, and gelatin.
- **Lacto-ovo vegetarians:** Do not eat meat, poultry, or fish, but do eat eggs and dairy products.
- **Lacto vegetarians:** Eat no meat, poultry, fish, or eggs, but do consume dairy products.
- **Ovo vegetarians:** Eat no meat, poultry, fish, or dairy products, but do eat eggs.
- **Partial vegetarians:** Avoid meat but may eat fish (pesco-vegetarian, pescatarian) or poultry (pollo-vegetarian).

Whatever the reason, the best way to eat for optimal health is to think like a vegan and eat your veggies! They are filling and full of fiber. When I work with a vegan or vegetarian, I typically ask what kind of vegan or vegetarian diet they follow. There is a large disparity between a vegan who eats mostly vegetables and plant proteins to one who eats mostly processed foods, large quantities of fruit, and pasta. I have counseled people who've come to me with complaints of weight gain and fatigue—and I am not surprised when they tell me they're eating the latter diet type. Cookies, French fries, soda, bread, pasta, and candy are some of the vegan options that I see consumed regularly by vegans and vegetarians. Eating that way is not something I recommend for anyone, especially vegans and vegetarians, as it is imperative for everyone to obtain their nutrients through good whole foods, so they don't have to worry about deficiencies.

VEGAN IS BEST FOR

A Vegan FoodFrame can improve heart health and contribute to a higher daily intake of fiber and micronutrients for those who follow it. There are numerous published studies, including the well-known China Study by Dr. Colin Campbell, that correlate cancer and heart disease with a diet high in animal protein and dairy.[7] I have seen vegans thrive and fail on this type of diet. Most of the outcome is dependent on the type of FoodFrame you adhere to (which I will elaborate on later) and your health status (what issues you are having at the time).

Whether for ethical, environmental, health, religious, or other reasons, I urge you and everyone else to fill 60-80 percent of your plate with greens or vegetables, and the remaining 20-40 percent should be nutrient-dense whole foods. Vegetables contain protein but in high numbers. If you consume enough of the recommended vegetables and other plant proteins such as legumes and nuts, you will be getting adequate amounts of protein.

Plant Foods and Fiber

Fiber is really the key here, especially as it's only found in plant foods. Fiber is a type of carbohydrate that

---

[7] Colin Campbell: The China Study- Animal protein and dairy and it's connection to cancer and heart disease. https://en.wikipedia.org/wiki/The_China_Study
The China Study examines the link between the consumption of animal products (including dairy) and chronic illnesses such as coronary heart disease, diabetes, breast cancer, prostate cancer, and bowel cancer.[4] The authors conclude that people who eat a predominantly whole-food, vegan diet—avoiding animal products as a main source of nutrition, including beef, pork, poultry, fish, eggs, cheese, and milk, and reducing their intake of processed foods and refined carbohydrates—will escape, reduce, or reverse the development of numerous diseases. They write that "eating foods that contain any cholesterol above 0 mg is unhealthy."[5]

your body does not digest; it provides no nutritional value but is essential for optimal health. There are three main forms of fiber: soluble fiber, insoluble fiber, and fermentable fiber:

- **Soluble fiber** dissolves in water and slows down digestion. It assists with lowering your cholesterol and blood sugar levels.
- **Insoluble fiber** will not dissolve in water, adds bulk to your stool, and passes through your digestive system more quickly. Basically, it prevents constipation.
- **Fermentable fiber** can originate from both categories, but it comes more often from soluble fibers. Fermented fibers help increase the healthy bacteria in your colon.

Fiber's role and its many health benefits include:

- Escorting toxins out of the body
- Feeding healthy gut bacteria
- Increasing the absorption of magnesium
- Lowering the risk of cardiovascular diseases and stroke
- Providing support in controlling systemic inflammation
- Reducing cholesterol
- Regulating digestion
- Regulating hunger hormones
- Slowing the release of insulin, preventing Type 2 diabetes
- Supporting weight loss

Fiber Requirements

According to the American Heart Association, fiber requirements for adults are roughly 25 grams daily. Women need 25 grams per day, men may need up to 38 grams, and children up to 18 years of age may need 14-31 grams daily. Sadly, most Americans are only getting an average of 16 grams per day.

The dramatic decrease of fiber consumption in American diets over the last 50 years is staggering. The shift from fiber-rich foods to refined carbohydrates--along with a significant increase in sugar consumption--has paralleled the increase in cardiovascular disease, Type 2 diabetes, and obesity. Vegans or vegetarians should find it easy to attain the required amount of fiber, but many do not because they're eating the wrong kinds of foods.

High and Low-Containing Fiber Foods

High Fiber

1 cup avocado	10 grams of fiber
1 cup broccoli, boiled	5 grams of fiber
1 cup lentils, boiled	15.5 grams of fiber
1 cup pistachios, raw	13 grams of fiber
1 cup raspberries	8 grams of fiber

Low Fiber

1 cup cantaloupe	1.6 grams of fiber
1 cup long-grain white rice	0.6 grams of fiber
1 cup watermelon	0.6 grams of fiber
1 slice white bread	0.8 grams of fiber
1 cup white mushrooms	0.7 grams of fiber

SIDEBAR – Shurbhi's Story

Shurbhi was adorable, with a clipped English accent and large, expressive eyes. But she came into my office with her concerned husband because she was insatiably hungry and had a serious addiction to sugar. They had left their Indian families and home in England for a career move to California shortly after she was diagnosed with psoriatic arthritis and psoriasis. For years, Shurbhi had experienced extreme fatigue (leading to daily afternoon naps), joint pain, bloating, and skin sensitivity. The doctors had prescribed steroids and anti-inflammatory drugs, with little success. She wanted to lose weight, have her food cravings go away, and feel better.

Shurbhi was raised in a traditional vegan family, primarily eating grains, beans, and gluten along with vegetables. I was a bit challenged in reducing her inflammation due to all the lectins in the grains and beans, along with naan, a traditional Indian bread, being her staple. I ordered my usual battery of blood and stool tests and immediately placed her on a vegan detox for 21 days along with a protocol of anti-inflammatory supplements to match a vegan FoodFrame, including more vegetables and less grains and legumes. We completely eliminated gluten and sugar and focused on nuts and seeds for protein, good quality fats, and I made sure the grains and legumes she did eat were pressure-cooked or soaked prior to eating to decrease the lectin load. Since good fats curb sugar cravings, her need for sweets diminished right away, and being satiated meant she could curb her habit of mindlessly snacking. We incorporated lots of anti-inflammatory spices like turmeric and ginger.

After just a few weeks, Shurbhi had so much more energy that she no longer needed her afternoon naps, and her need for medication decreased. After a month, her pain completely disappeared, and she lost enough weight to hit her target goal. Shurbhi loved to cook and created amazing vegetable dishes that she looked forward to eating with her family.

WHO SHOULD AVOID THE VEGAN DIET

If you have digestive issues or illnesses such as ulcerative colitis, Crohn's disease, irritable bowel syndrome, or diverticulitis, you may need to eat a low-fiber diet. If so, I would recommend the AIP Protocol as a better fit, but if you insist on being vegan or vegetarian and experience a flare-up, then I would absolutely recommend sticking to low-fiber foods until it passes.

Through my own experience being a vegan and pescatarian, I lived through what a diet high in legumes and grains can cause--my blood sugar continued to rise and my thyroid was failing even though I wasn't eating processed foods. You need to be aware of the pitfalls of going vegan as well as its benefits. Again, much depends on what type of vegan or vegetarian you are.

When Being Vegan Can Harm You

I see many vegans and vegetarians in my practice. It pains me that most of them are sick and not thriving. Unknowingly, they may not be getting enough of the essential nutrients we require from our food, which can lead to serious health consequences:

- The biggest problem is Vitamin B12, which can only be found in animal foods, particularly meat. You can get a little bit from nutritional yeast, but not in the amount your body needs. Iron obtained from meat is more readily absorbed than the iron found in plants. For example, you would have to eat an exceptionally large amount of spinach to get the same amount of iron in a much smaller amount of meat. I do recommend supplementing with a quality methylcobalamin B complex vitamin with ample B12.
- Zinc is a critical mineral that is needed for many processes of the body, as it's the precursor to the synthesis of digestive enzymes, proteins, and DNA. A severe zinc deficiency causes damage to DNA from oxidative stress. Zinc boosts the immune system's ability to fight off bacteria and viruses, and is critical during pregnancy, infancy, and childhood for proper development. Zinc is found in small quantities in vegetables, but when eating more whole grains, seeds, beans, and legumes, the phytic acid in those foods reduces the absorption of zinc. This can unwittingly lead to deficiencies.
- Omegas-3 fatty acids are comprised of DHA (docosahexaenoic acid) and EPA (eicosatetraenoic acid) which are essential for many different functions, but particularly for brain and heart health, cholesterol, and triglyceride management, blood pressure regulation, eye health, and depression and anxiety. They are also a wonderful anti-inflammatory. The only source is from fish or algae, but vegans can get ALA (alpha-linolenic acid) from nuts, seeds, and soy; it converts into EPA and DHA--but not very efficiently. The conversion rate ranges from 8-10 percent, which usually isn't high enough to give you optimal benefits. I recommend supplementing with a fish oil, which some vegans are open to doing.
- Blood sugar dysregulation can easily occur if your diet consists of mostly processed foods, high-sugar fruits, or other foods high in carbohydrates and sugar. It is absolutely possible to become a Type 2 diabetic from eating these foods on a regular basis. Fiber, along with protein and fat, is what slows that spike of sugar—fiber is not found in sufficient quantities in highly processed and sugar-laden foods.
- Weight gain is quite common amongst vegans and vegetarians. Some of my vegan clients

are very thin because they don't know how to sustain their caloric needs; others are very heavy because their hunger drives them to eat junk or a lot of calorie-dense foods that are nutritious, like nuts, but should not be eaten in large quantities. These clients often sustain themselves on a diet with super-high levels of carbs that cause blood sugar dysregulation, weight gain, and fatigue. These negate the health benefits many people are looking for when they go vegan.

If you go vegan, it is critical to keep track of your sugar and carbohydrate intake—by now you know that sugar, or foods that turn into sugar, makes people fat. When your pancreas pumps out insulin, it doesn't matter if it's triggered by a mango or a Twinkie--your body will respond by trying to get the sugar into your cells and storing the excess as fat.

Another possible precaution is the potential amount of soy consumption. Soy is an abundant source of protein and a staple for many vegans and vegetarians. One cup of boiled soybeans contains a whopping 29 grams of protein, so it leads the race as a more-than-viable source of plant-based protein. Unfermented food uses of soybeans include soymilk, tofu, and tofu skin. Fermented soy foods include soy sauce (tamari, shoyu, and teriyaki), fermented bean paste, nattō, and tempeh. It can also be found in many meat alternatives such as vegan/vegetarian burgers, sausages, bacon, chicken, and hotdogs. Dairy alternatives like cheese and yogurt can be soy-based as well. Soy lecithin and soy protein isolate are found in a variety of foods as an additive. Soybeans are made into miso, crispy soy nuts, and enjoyed in many Japanese restaurants in the form of edamame, eaten right out of the pod. Soybean oil is commonly used in many processed foods and supplements. Animal feed and infant formula is often soy-based.

While soy sounds like the perfect food as it's high in protein, low in calories and carbs, and contains a decent amount of fiber, vitamins, and minerals, it does come with plenty of controversy. Soy has been touted to reduce some cancers and osteoporosis risk, enhance fertility, and alleviate menopause symptoms--but it has also been linked to decrease thyroid function, gastric issues, imbalanced estrogen and testosterone, reduced absorbability of zinc and iron, and soy allergy. Soy carries isoflavones which essentially mimic estrogen; this can be beneficial for someone low in estrogen, but harmful for those who don't need excess estrogen.

In addition, 94 percent of the soy supply in the United States and Canada consists of genetically modified organisms (GMO), meaning that the soybean has been artificially engineered in a laboratory from its original and natural state to lessen the need for herbicides or pesticides. But since the herbicides and pesticides don't always work as intended, and insects can become resistant to them, more chemicals can be needed to counteract this resistance, leaving even more chemical residue in or on the plants. There are 64 countries that require GMO labeling. The US has recently passed the DARK ACT that requires some, but not all, foods that contain GMOs to be labeled by 2022.

It is a bit too early to have studies that prove the safety or harm from eating GMO foods, but there is a lot of speculation about the dangers. I always recommend that you buy crops and food without GMOs, as I believe we should be eating food in its original form, the way it was intended for your body to process and absorb nutrients. If choosing to eat soy and soy products, I highly recommend you choose non-GMO sources, in addition to organic soy.

VEGAN FOODS TO ENJOY

Plant-Based Proteins

Hemp tofu, seitan, soy, soy tofu, tempeh

Leafy Vegetables

*Unlimited

Arugula, beet greens, Bok choy, broccoli rabe, Brussels sprouts, cabbage, carrot tops, celery, chicory, collard greens, cress, dandelion greens, endive, kale - all varieties, lettuce - all varieties, mustard greens, Napa cabbage, purslane, radicchio, sorrel, spinach, spirulina, swiss chard, tatsoi, turnip greens, watercress

Non-starchy Vegetables

Artichoke, asparagus, broccoli, cauliflower, celery root, fennel, rhubarb, squash blossoms

Vegetables

Cucumber, squash (all varieties), pumpkin, yellow summer squash, zucchini

Allium-family Vegetables

Chive, garlic, leek, onion, scallion, shallot, wild leek

Roots, Tubers, and Bulb Vegetables

Arrowroot, bamboo shoot, beet, burdock, carrot, cassava, celeriac, daikon, ginger, glucomannan, horseradish and root, Jerusalem artichoke, jicama, kohlrabi, lotus root, parsnip, radish, rutabaga, sweet potato, taro, Tiger nuts, turnip, wasabi, water chestnut, yam (yam noodles), yucca

Nightshades or Spices Derived from Nightshades

*Omit or limit if Autoimmune (see Chapter 5)

Ashwagandha, capsicums/peppers, chili pepper flakes, chili powder, curry, cayenne pepper, jalapeno, paprika, pepinos, peppers (bell, chipotle, hot, red, and sweet) and pimentos; cape gooseberries, eggplant, goji berries (wolfberries), potatoes (sweet potatoes and yams are not nightshades and are okay), sweet plantains, tomatoes (all varieties)

Grains and Grain-Like Foods

Amaranth, barley, buckwheat, bulgur, corn, farro, millet, oats/oatmeal, quinoa, rice, wild rice, rye, sorghum, spelt, teff, wheat (all varieties, including einkorn and semolina)

Sea Vegetables

Arame, dulse, hijiki, kombu, nori, wakame

Vegetable-like Fruits

Avocado, bitter melon, chayote, cucumber, okra, olives, plantain, persimmons, pumpkin, squash (all varieties), winter melon, zucchini

Berries

Acai, blackberry, blueberry, cranberry, currant, elderberry, gooseberry, grapes (all varieties), lingonberry, mulberry, raspberry, strawberry

Rosaceae-family Fruits

Apple, apricot, cherry, nectarine, peach, pear, plum, quince, rosehip

Melons

Cantaloupe, honeydew, horned melon, melon pear, Persian melon, watermelon, winter melon

Citrus-family Fruits

Clementine, grapefruit, kumquat, lemon, lime, orange, pomelo, tangelo, tangerine, yuzu

Tropical Fruits

Acerola, banana, chayote, cherimoya, coconut, date, dragon fruit, durian, fig, guava, jackfruit, kiwi, loquat, lychee, mango, mangosteen, papaya, passion fruit, pawpaw, persimmon, pineapple, plantain, pomegranate, star fruit, tamarind

Edible Fungi/Mushrooms

Chanterelle, cremini, morel, oyster, porcini, portobello, shiitake, truffle

Legumes

Adzuki beans, black beans, black-eyed peas, butter beans, calico beans, cannellini beans, chickpeas (garbanzo beans), fava beans (broad beans), great northern beans, green beans, Italian beans, kidney beans, lentils, lima beans, mung beans, navy beans, peanuts, peas, pinto beans, runner beans, soybeans (including edamame, tofu, tempeh, other soy products, and soy isolates, such as soy lecithin), split peas, sprouts (all varieties), sugar snap peas

Plant Fats

Algae oil, avocado oil (cold-pressed), canola oil, coconut oil, extra virgin olive oil (cold-pressed), MCT (medium chain triglycerides) oil, palm shortening, perilla oil, red palm oil, rice bran oil, sesame oil, walnut oil

Processed Vegetable Oils

Permitted but not recommended

Canola oil (rapeseed oil), corn oil, cottonseed oil, grapeseed oil, palm kernel oil, peanut oil, safflower oil, soybean oil, sunflower oil, partially and hydrogenated oils

Nuts/Nut Butters and Nut Oils

Almonds, Brazil, cashews, chestnuts, hazelnuts, macadamia, pistachios, peanuts, pecans, pine nuts, walnuts

Seeds and Seed Butters

Chia, sesame, flax, hemp, poppy, psyllium, pumpkin, sunflower seeds

Dairy

*Watch for ingredients that contain casein

All yogurts, cheeses, spreads, creams, ice creams made from almond, cashew, coconut, hemp, oat, soy, or rice milks.

Probiotic Foods

Kombucha (unless sweetened with honey), kvass, non-dairy kefir, non-dairy yogurt, fermented fruits and vegetables, sauerkraut

Herbs and Spices

Allspice, anise, annatto, basil leaf, bay leaf, black caraway, cardamom, celery seed, chamomile, Chinese five-spice powder, chervil, chives, cilantro, coriander, cinnamon, cloves, cumin, curry powder, dill, fennel seed, fennel leaf, fenugreek, garlic, ginger, garam masala, juniper, kaffir lime leaf, lavender, lemongrass, mace, marjoram leaf, mustard, nutmeg, onion powder, oregano leaf, parsley, pepper, peppermint, poppy, rosemary, saffron, sage, savory leaf, sea or Himalayan salt, spearmint, tarragon, thyme, truffles, turmeric, vanilla

Flavorings

*Watch for added ingredients

Apple cider vinegar, balsamic vinegar, capers, carob powder, coconut aminos (a soy sauce substitute), coconut concentrate, coconut milk, coconut water vinegar, fruit and vegetable juice (in moderation), organic jams and chutneys (in moderation), miso, red wine vinegar, soy sauce, truffle oil (made with olive oil), white wine vinegar

Flours

Almond, arrowroot, cassava, chestnut, coconut, garbanzo, grapeseed, green banana, hazelnut, pastry flour, semolina, sesame, soy, sweet potato, tapioca, tiger nut, wheat, whole wheat

Added Sugars

Agave, agave nectar, barley malt, barley malt syrup, beet sugar, brown rice syrup, brown sugar, cane crystals, cane juice, cane sugar, raw cane sugar, evaporated cane juice, and dehydrated cane juice, corn sweetener, corn syrup, and corn syrup solids, crystalline fructose, date sugar, demerara sugar, dextrin, dextrose, fructose, high-fructose corn syrup, fruit juice, fruit juice concentrate, glucose, glucose solids, golden syrup, invert sugar, jaggery, malt syrup, maltodextrin, maltose, muscovado sugar, palm sugar, raw sugar, refined sugar, rice bran syrup, rice syrup, saccharose, sorghum syrup, sucanat, sucrose, syrup, treacle, turbinado sugar, yacon syrup

Sweeteners

Allulose, stevia, inulin, yacon, monk fruit (Luo Han Guo), dark chocolate (check ingredients)

Sugar Alcohols

Erythritol, mannitol, sorbitol, xylitol

Non-nutritive Sweeteners

Permitted but not recommended

Acesulfame potassium, aspartame (Equal), neotame, saccharin (Sweet 'n Low), stevia, sucralose (Splenda)

Processed Food Chemicals and Ingredients

Permitted but not recommended

Acrylamides, any ingredient with an unrecognizable chemical name, artificial and natural flavors, artificial food color, autolyzed protein, brominated vegetable oil, caramel, emulsifiers (carrageenan, cellulose gum, guar gum, lecithin), hydrolyzed vegetable protein, monosodium glutamate, nitrates or nitrites (naturally occurring are okay), olestra, phosphoric acid, propylene glycol, textured vegetable protein, trans fats (partially hydrogenated vegetable oil, hydrogenated oil), yeast extract

Beverages

Water (club, mineral, reverse osmosis, seltzer, soda, sparkling [without natural flavors, sweeteners, and additives], spring); almond milk (unsweetened), coconut milk, coconut water (in moderation), coffee (decaf and caffeinated), electrolyte drinks, energy drinks, green juices (freshly squeezed), hemp milk (unsweetened), oat milk, rice milk, teas (black, green, or herbal), sodas (diet and regular), sports drinks, soy milk, yerba mate

Alcohol

Beer (most beers are good except for some British ones), bourbon, gin, rum, schnapps, tequila, vodka, whiskey (Canadian, Irish, Scotch, Tennessee), wine (avoid ones made with egg whites, casein, gelatin, isinglass, chitosan)

VEGAN FOODS TO AVOID

Meat

Includes broth and collagen

Cattle (beef, veal), deer (venison), goat, hare, pig (pork), rabbit, sheep (lamb, mutton), wild game (buffalo/bison, boar, elk)

Poultry

Includes broth and collagen

Chicken, duck, goose, grouse, guinea hen, ostrich, pheasant, quail, turkey

Fish

Includes broth and collagen

Anchovy, arctic char, bass, bonito, carp, catfish, cod, eel, gar, haddock, hake, halibut, herring, mackerel, mahi-mahi, marlin, monkfish, perch, pollock, salmon, sardine, snapper, sole, swordfish, tilapia, trout, tuna (fresh ahi or yellowfin, or canned), turbot, walleye

Shellfish

Includes broth and collagen

Clams, crab, crawfish, lobster, mussels, octopus, oysters, scallops, shrimp, squid

Eggs

Chicken, duck, goose, quail, including fish eggs/caviar

Animal Fats

Bacon fat, butter (grass-fed), ghee, goat butter, lard, leaf lard (fat from pig), pan drippings, poultry fat, schmaltz (chicken or goose fat), strutto (clarified pork fat), tallow (from beef, lamb, or mutton)

Probiotic Foods

Fermented meat or fish

Dairy

Buttermilk, cheeses (cow, cream cheese, goat, high-fat, low-fat, sheep), cow's milk, cow's milk yogurt, cream (crème fraiche, dairy creamer, half and half, heavy, sour, whipped) curds, dairy protein isolates, goat and sheep kefir, whey-protein isolate

Added Proteins and Sugars

Casein, gelatin, honey, lactose, whey (isolate and concentrate)

Beverages

Check ingredients

Dairy-based drinks (kefir, coffees, boba)

Alcohol

Beer (most beers are good except for some British ones), champagne, wine (avoid ones made with egg whites, casein, gelatin, isinglass, chitosan)

LIFE AFTER VEGAN

A vegan lifestyle is certainly doable for the long term, but you need to be vigilant about your food choices and consider being a partial vegan if you have trouble sticking to the plan. If so, partial vegans can easily stick to this eating plan for life, as there are so many vegetarian options available, no matter what kind of food you like. Some vegans and vegetarians are open to animal nutrients such as fish oils and collagen. These are derived from animals, but they are not the animal flesh and the benefits are so impactful, especially as there are virtually no vegan substitutes. I urge you to make every meal count and avoid the high-carbohydrate foods that are so convenient on the vegan and vegetarian lifestyle.

As you read earlier in this chapter, you need to ensure you get enough essential micronutrients:

- B12 is sourced mainly from animal protein, so if you are a strict vegan, I recommend supplementing with a quality methylated B vitamin complex. Small amounts of B12 can be found in nutritional yeast and some varieties of mushrooms (dried shitake or Lion's Mane) and algae but I encourage you to track your levels when you do blood work. It can be common for strict vegans to have a B12 anemia which can cause a cascade of dysregulation. Fortified processed foods can have some B12 but as you know by now, that is not something I highly recommend. Many vegetarians will eat eggs which, if consumed weekly, can sometimes be enough of a B12 source.
- Zinc has several animal and plant sources. Legumes such as garbanzos, lentils and most beans contain a substantial amount of zinc. Pumpkin seeds are another great source and I personally put a tablespoon of them in my morning shake. Other sources are nuts, potatoes, grains like wheat, quinoa, rice and oats along with dark chocolate.
- Omega 3 fatty acids are ideally sourced from fish oil, but you can get a little from algae. Again, if not opposed to taking a fish oil, I highly recommend it as the number of benefits cannot be found in equal amounts from vegan sources.
- Iron is extremely important! Avoiding any type of anemia is critical for optimal health as it can affect other systems. Without question, meat or animal protein is the ideal source, but you can obtain it from plants such as legumes, nuts, seeds, spinach, broccoli, and dried fruits like apricots, raisins, and prunes - all are great plant sources of iron. Again, I highly recommend you keep an eye out for iron deficiency.

RECIPES - VEGAN

Pumpkin Pie Shake

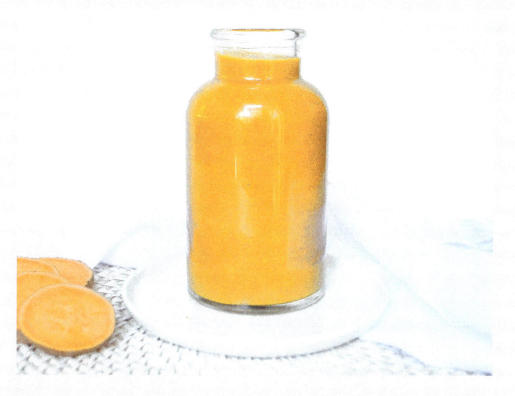

🍴 Ingredients:

¼ cup raw or roasted almonds
1 teaspoon chia seeds
1 cup water or coconut milk, unsweetened
2 handfuls of greens (spinach, kale, etc.)

½ – 1 cup pumpkin puree
1 tablespoon pumpkin pie spice
2 teaspoon cinnamon
1 handful ice cubes

🍴 Instructions:

Place all ingredients into a blender and blend until well combined.

Serves 1

Risa Groux, CN

Blueberry Breakfast Cookies

🍴 Ingredients:

2 ripe bananas
2 ½ cups gluten-free rolled oats
1 cup cashew butter
½ cup sunflower seeds
¼ cup honey or maple syrup
1 teaspoon vanilla extract
½ teaspoon ground cinnamon
¼ teaspoon sea salt
1 cup fresh or frozen blueberries

🍴 Instructions:

Preheat oven to 325 degrees. Line a baking sheet with parchment paper and set aside.

1. Add all ingredients until well combined.
2. Roll dough into balls and place on a cookie sheet. Flatten with the bottom of a glass.
3. Bake for 20 minutes or until lightly browned on the bottom and sides.
4. Cool for 5 minutes and serve.

Stays fresh in the refrigerator for up to a week.

Makes about 12 cookies

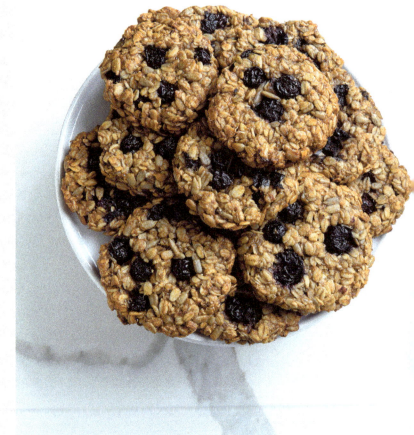

Garlic Rosemary White Bean Dip

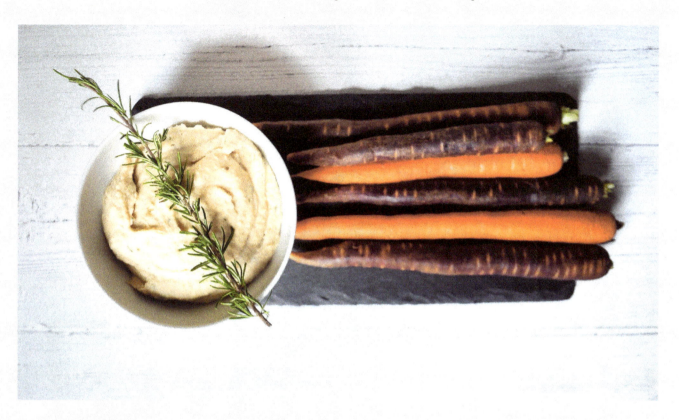

🍴 Ingredients:

3 cups cooked white beans (cannellini, navy, or great northern)
¼ cup extra-virgin olive oil
1 large lemon, juiced (about ¼ cup)

1 to 2 cloves garlic, peeled and coarsely chopped
1 tablespoon chopped fresh rosemary
1 teaspoon sea salt

🍴 Instructions:

Place all ingredients in a food processor or blender and process until smooth and creamy. Garnish with rosemary.

Serves 10-12

Green Gazpacho

🍴 Ingredients:

1 pint yellow grape tomatoes (approximately 2 cups)
1 English cucumber, skin on
1 fennel bulb, trimmed, core removed
2 celery stalks
2 scallions
½ jalapeño, seeded
2 garlic cloves
1-2 large handful(s) of baby spinach
1 bunch basil (a large handful or two)
1-2 cups water (depending on how thick you like it)
2 ripe avocados
2 limes, juiced
1 tablespoon white balsamic vinegar
2 tablespoons olive oil
Sea salt and pepper to taste

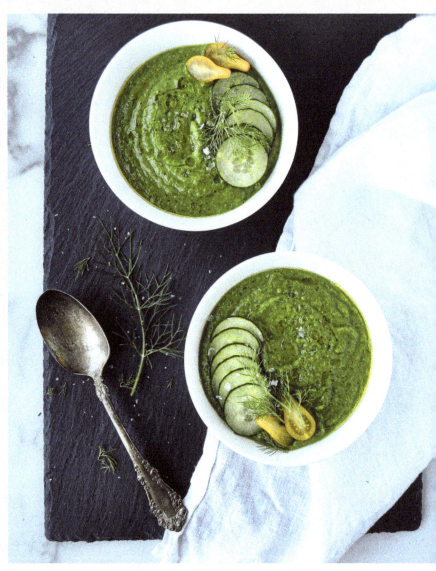

🍴 Instructions:

1. Finely chop cucumber and tomatoes in a food processor and put in large bowl.
2. In the same food processor, finely chop the fennel, celery, scallions, jalapeño, and garlic, and add to the bowl with the cucumber and tomatoes.
3. Add the spinach and basil to the food processor and chop. Add to the bowl.
4. Add water and stir to combine all the ingredients.
5. Add about 2 cups of the mixture back into the food processor with the avocado, lime juice, vinegar, olive oil, salt, and pepper. Process until smooth.
6. Return mixture to the bowl and stir well to combine all ingredients.
7. Taste for additional seasoning.
8. Chill for a couple hours prior to serving.

Serves 6

Autumn Kale Salad

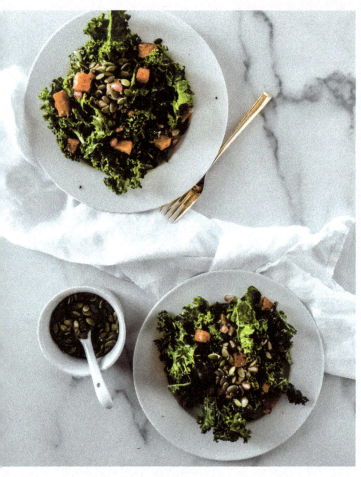

Ingredients:

Salad:

1 large butternut squash (about 3 pounds), peeled cut into ¾" cubes
4 teaspoons extra virgin olive oil
½ tablespoon cinnamon
Sea salt and freshly ground black pepper, to taste
1 ½ pounds Tuscan kale (about 2-3 large bunches), stemmed, leaves thinly sliced into strips
½ cup raw pumpkin seeds (pepitas)
1 cup pomegranate seeds (1 large pomegranate)

Dressing:

½ cup extra virgin olive oil
1 whole head garlic
¼ cup fresh lemon juice (from 1 large lemon)
2 teaspoons raw honey (optional)
2 tablespoons Dijon mustard
1 tablespoon finely chopped shallot

Instructions:

Preheat oven to 350 degrees.

1. Toss cubed butternut squash in a bowl with 4 teaspoons olive oil, cinnamon, sea salt, and pepper until well coated. Place on a baking sheet and cook butternut squash until soft and slightly brown (approximately 30-40 minutes). Remove from the oven and let cool.
2. Make the salad dressing by putting all ingredients into a blender or mini chopper, blending well.
3. Place kale and butternut squash into a bowl. Top with pumpkin seeds and pomegranate seeds. Drizzle the dressing over top and serve.

Serves 4-6

Beet Quinoa Cauliflower

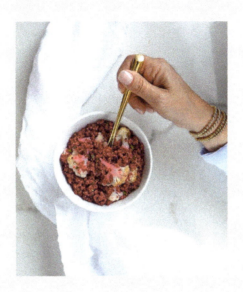

Ingredients:

1 small red beet, roasted
¼ cup almond or coconut milk
1 cup raw quinoa
½ cauliflower, roasted

½ cup Italian parsley, roughly chopped
¼ cup olive oil
Sea salt and pepper to taste

Instructions:

1. Wash beet and roast in the oven in 375F oven for 45 minutes. Roast cauliflower in the same oven but in a different pan for approximately 45 minutes.
2. Boil 2 cups of water or bone broth in a pan. Add quinoa and simmer for 15 minutes until liquid is absorbed. Pour cooked quinoa in a bowl and add roasted cauliflower.
3. Remove the skin from the roasted beet, place in a mini chopper/blender and add nut milk. Blend well but don't liquify the mixture. Add more nut milk if needed.

Pour the beet mixture over the quinoa and mix until all quinoa is red. Add parsley, olive oil, salt, and pepper.

Serves 4-6

Vegetable Tikka Masala

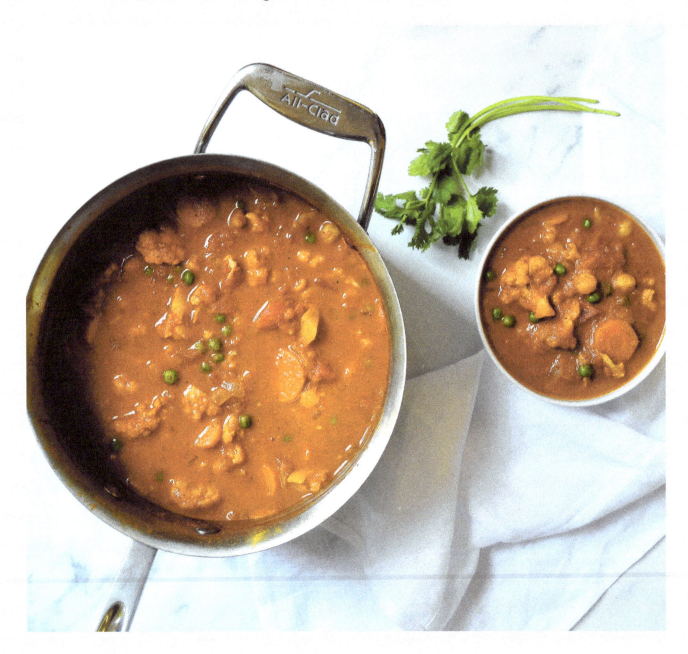

Ingredients:

- 1 large yellow onion (½ for sauce, ½ finely chopped and reserved)
- 2 cloves of garlic
- 1-inch fresh ginger, peeled
- 10 sprigs fresh cilantro, plus more for garnish (rough chop)
- 2 tablespoons olive oil, divided
- ½ teaspoon cumin
- ½ teaspoon turmeric
- ¼ teaspoon ground cinnamon
- 1 teaspoon paprika
- 1 teaspoon sea salt
- 1 ½ teaspoons garam masala
- 15 oz canned plum tomatoes, with the juices
- 1 15 oz can tomato sauce
- 1 15 oz can full fat coconut cream or milk
- ½ head cauliflower, chopped into bite sized pieces
- 3 large carrots, peeled and finely chopped
- 1 15 oz can chickpeas, drained and rinsed
- Additional chopped cilantro for garnish

Instructions:

1. In a food processor, combine half of the onion, garlic, ginger, cilantro, and 1 tablespoon of olive oil. Blend until smooth about 1 minute. Set aside.
2. In a large skillet, heat the remaining olive oil over medium heat. Add in the reserved chopped onion and spices, stir to combine and cook gently for 10 minutes. Add the plum tomatoes (with the liquid), tomato sauce, half a can of coconut milk or cream, add the blended onion and cilantro sauce. Cook for an additional 5 minutes over medium heat. Add in the cauliflower and carrots and bring to a simmer. Simmer for 20 minutes.
3. Once the veggies are tender, add in chickpeas and the remaining coconut milk or cream. Stir to combine and let cook for 5 more minutes.

Optional: You can add additional veggies like broccoli and Brussels sprouts.

Serve over brown rice, quinoa or millet.

Serves 8

Vegan Protein Bowl

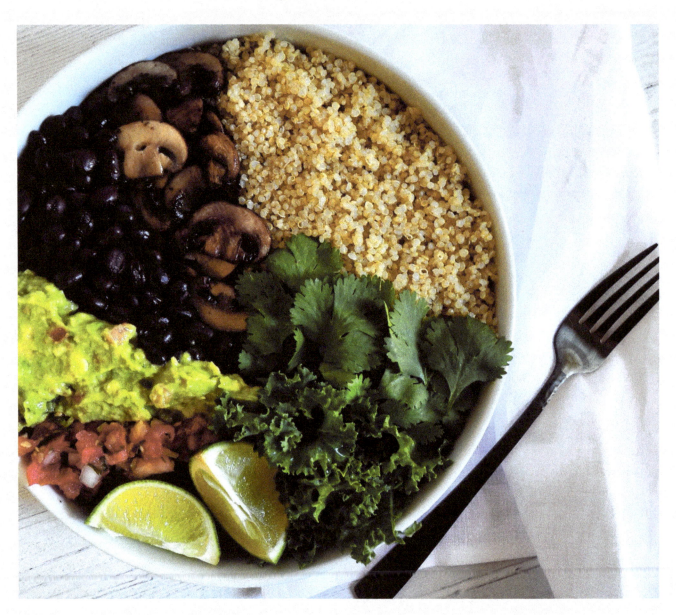

Ingredients:

For Salad:
1-1 ½ cups romaine lettuce, torn
1-1 ½ cups cooked quinoa
1 cup black beans, rinsed and drained
1 cup zucchini, sliced and quartered

1 cup yellow onion, diced
1 ½ - 2 cups kale or spinach
1 cup mushrooms, sliced (can sub another veggie)
Sea salt to taste

For salsa:
2 ripe tomatoes
¼ cup white onion, diced
1 jalapeno, deseeded and diced

¼ - ½ cup cilantro, chopped
½ lime, juiced
Sea salt to taste

For guacamole:
1-1½ ripe avocados
¼ -½ cup lime juice
Sea salt to taste

Instructions:

1. Cook quinoa in water or vegetable stock and set aside.
2. Heat the black beans and set them aside.
3. Wash and dry romaine leaves then tear into bite size pieces and set aside.
4. Sauté onions, zucchini, kale (or spinach) and mushrooms and set aside.
5. Remove seeds and juice from the tomatoes keeping the skins intact. Cut the tomatoes into small dice and place in a bowl.
6. Dice onion and jalapeno and place together in a bowl along with the chopped cilantro. Mix together and add lime juice and salt to taste.
7. Mash the avocados in a separate bowl and add 1 to 2 tablespoons of salsa. Add a little squeeze of lime and salt if needed.
8. Layer the bowl starting with romaine lettuce followed by quinoa, black beans, and sautéed vegetables. Top with a dollop of guacamole and salsa.

Garnish with cilantro.

Serves 4-6

Strawberry Cheesecake Bars

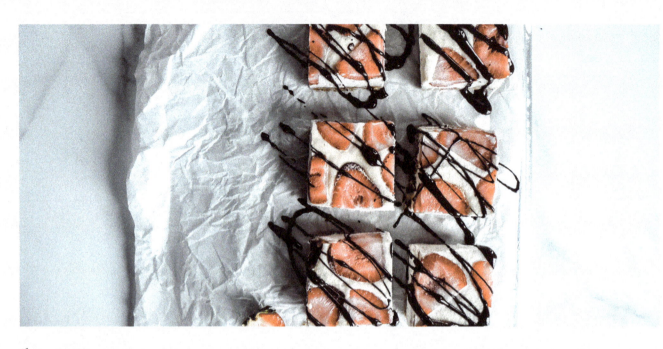

🍴 Ingredients:

Crust:

¾ cup raw cashews
¼ cup almond flour
4 medjool dates, pitted
2 tablespoons coconut oil
¼ teaspoon sea salt

Cheesecake:

2 cups raw cashews, soaked in cold water
½ cup canned coconut milk, shake to blend well
¼ cup coconut oil, melted and cooled
⅓ cup pure maple syrup or monk fruit flavored with maple syrup
2 tablespoons fresh lemon juice
1 tablespoon vanilla extract or 1 teaspoon vanilla bean powder
2 cups organic strawberries, washed and halved
¼ cup dark chocolate, melted

🍴 Instructions:

Line an 8x8" pan with parchment paper and grease well with coconut oil. Set aside.

Crust:
1. Add the raw cashews, almond flour, pitted dates, coconut oil, and salt to a food processor or high-powered blender and pulse until it comes together into a crumbly and sticky dough, with small bits remaining. Be careful not to over process.
2. Press the dough evenly along the bottom of the prepared pan. Use the back of a spatula to flatten evenly.
3. Place in the fridge while making the filling.

Cheesecake:
1. In the same food processor or blender, combine all the filling ingredients except the strawberries and blend for approximately 2 minutes until the mixture is smooth and creamy. Scrape down the sides if needed.
2. If using a blender, you may need to add a drop more coconut milk or lemon juice to get it smooth.

Assembly:
1. Remove pan from fridge and pour the cheesecake over the crust. Smooth out the top to make sure it's even and tap the pan against the counter a few times to release any air bubbles. Once everything is settled and even, press the strawberry halves randomly into the cheesecake with the inside of the strawberry facing up.
2. Place in the freezer to firm up for at least 3 hours before cutting.
3. Run a knife under hot water to warm it up before cutting the bars with the still hot but dried knife.
4. Let thaw at room temperature for 15-20 minutes.
5. While waiting for the bars to cool, melt the chocolate (see note) in double broiler or microwave and drizzle over the bars before serving.

Makes 16 bars

Note: Using a double boiler, fill the bottom pot slightly less than halfway with water and place the chocolate in the top pot. On low heat stir continuously until smooth, remove immediately. If you don't have a double broiler, you can use a regular pot and place a heatproof or glass bowl on top of the pot. Proceed the same way. Make sure the bowl does not touch the water but rather let the steam melt the chocolate. Either way, be careful not to overheat the chocolate as it will clump.

CHAPTER 8

THE LOW LECTIN FOODFRAME

All living organisms have two goals: survival and procreation. For those goals to be attainable, they need a way to defend themselves. When humans are in danger, they can flee, kick, bite, or scream. Plants have fewer options, obviously, so they evolved in a cunning way: they use proteins called lectins as a first line of defense.

Lectins are carbohydrate-binding proteins found in many foods, but primarily plant foods. They fall under the category of anti-nutrients, which means they can block the absorption of nutrients. The purpose of lectins is to preserve the germ/seed of a plant and deflect insects, pests, and microorganisms to ensure the plant's survival. In essence, they're a hard shell that surrounds the germ/seed of the plant and are strong enough to remain intact when we digest them. (Remember, their goal is to survive and procreate!) Lectins are abundant in raw legumes, especially in the part of the seed that becomes the leaves when the plant sprouts; grains; some dairy products; and a few vegetables known as nightshades. They may be the reason why you get very gassy when eating baked beans or hummus, or if you get painfully bloated after having pasta with tomato sauce.

Instead of being easily digestible, lectins can cause gas, bloating, weight gain, and inflammation, particularly for those with an imbalanced gut microbiome that produces a decreased number of digestive enzymes. If the stomach has low levels of acid, digestion is hindered making it exceptionally difficult to breakdown the lectins. The food then begins to putrefy and activates gasses to help break it down and move it through the digestive tract.

In addition, when you eat a plant food with a high level of lectins, such as a tomato, the lectins can go through the intestinal lining where, bit by bit they begin to eat away at the villi that protects the mucosal lining. Lectins and gluten can efficiently eat away at this thin and fragile lining and cause tight junctions, or little cracks in the intestinal wall, that allow undigested food (mostly proteins) and toxins to enter the blood system through the back door. This is called leaky gut or intestinal permeability. The body's immune system now sees these proteins and toxins as the enemy and creates antigens which turn into antibodies to attack the invaders. That is your immune system at work—but in this case it isn't ridding your body of a toxic invader like bacteria or a virus. It's responding to the food you just ate!

Lectins not only cause this damage but also impair the ability of cell regeneration, as they ignite your T regulatory (T Reg) cells to engage. We all have these cells that modulate our immune function, constantly patrolling to make sure your body's immune system is balanced and protected. When antibodies are produced, the T Reg cells kick into gear and create cytokines that ignite inflammation. That process is how cellular inflammation is created. You may feel perfectly fine when you eat these foods, but your body is in an ongoing state of attack. And when your body is in this state meal after meal, day after day, month after month, year after year, it begins to break down. This sets the stage for disease, which thrives in a state of systemic inflammation. Without proper nutrients to decrease inflammation, your body will stay in a cytokine storm, or a continuous state of inflammation that leaves you highly susceptible to viruses and disease. Removing lectins will alleviate the relentless attacks and therefore begin to heal your gut.

Some people can eat lectin-rich foods all their lives and not have any digestive or health issues at all. Many others will be victim to the lectins and, in addition to systemic inflammation, will gain weight, develop Irritable Bowel Syndrome (IBS), and likely attain autoimmune disorders caused by leaky gut syndrome. Studies all over the world are ongoing to pinpoint specifics and look for advanced treatments, but for now, the easiest way to treat this problem is to remove lectins from your diet. This has been shown to reduce these autoimmune disorders and, in some cases, reverse them.

Nightshades are particularly high in lectins and are usually concentrated in the seeds and skin of these foods. Nightshades are:

- Eggplants
- Goji berries
- Peppers (all kinds except black pepper)
- Potatoes (except yam and sweet potatoes)
- Tomatoes (all kinds)

In addition to nightshades, lectins can be found in high doses in almost all grains, legumes, squashes, and cucumber skin and seeds. Also try to avoid chia seeds along with cashews and peanuts as they are technically a legume, not a nut. All fruits are high in lectins with the exception of berries (when in season only), kiwi, and avocado.

Soaking, sprouting, or pressure-cooking grains and legumes will decrease lectin levels, and many people will enjoy those foods from time to time. Millet is a lovely nutty grain that is fairly low in lectins, which makes it the perfect substitute for quinoa. You should also enjoy many vegetables along with high-quality animal protein and good fats.

I recommend that you remove all nightshades and the foods listed above entirely when you go on the Low Lectin diet. Technically, you can remove the seeds and skin from tomatoes, peppers, cucumbers, or squashes to significantly decrease the lectin levels, but I would suggest you do this rarely for maximum results.

Some dairy is included in the Low Lectin FoodFrame as it contains a type of casein called A2 that is much easier to digest than A1 due to a difference in ratios of lactose and fatty acid, but the primary difference comes down to one differing amino acid. Casein are proteins that make up 80 % of the protein in dairy from cows. Certain cows of Western origin such as Holstein, and Jersey make A1 casein while others from Indian origin like Gir and Sahiwal make A2 casein. These are usually labeled and suggested for those who struggle with dairy. High-fat dairy does not typically contain casein, so it is included in the diet. It is estimated that two-thirds of the population is lactose intolerant, so I encourage most people to remove it from their diet. Once you remove it for a few weeks and then add it back, you may have a reaction. The vast amount of dairy we produce in the United States comes from animals who were fed growth hormones and given antibiotics; whatever dairy you consume from those animals gets into your body as well. This is partly why we are seeing children with precocious puberty, developing earlier than previous generations.

In addition, not having the necessary enzymes to break down lactose can cause stomach distress. Digestive enzymes are proteins that help break down food into macro and micronutrients so the body can use them for nourishment. Salivary enzymes are produced at the mere smell or thought of food; this is where the digestion process starts, in the mouth. Different types of enzymes break down different nutrients. The primary ones are amylase, which breaks down starches and carbohydrates; lipase, which breaks down fats; and protease, which breaks down proteins.

As we age, we produce and excrete fewer digestive enzymes. I remember my grandma used to say, "I can't eat that anymore," and as a child, I always wondered why. It was because she couldn't break down those foods any longer without experiencing stomach distress. And, in addition to age, other factors can contribute to loss of enzyme production: stress eats up our B vitamins which we need to produce enzymes; zinc and other vitamin deficiencies can cause problems, as can liver disease, pancreatic disease, and gastrointestinal diseases like Crohn's; and antibiotic use changes our gut microbiome and depletes its good bacteria.

I suggest taking a digestive enzyme supplement for most people over 50 years of age but will recommend them for people at any age dealing with heartburn and acid reflux—I see great results. Digestive enzymes can help with bloating, gas, diarrhea, heartburn, or acid reflux. If you have any type of gastrointestinal disease, it's always best to consult with your medical practitioner.

WHAT THE LOW LECTIN FOODFRAME IS BEST FOR

Going on a Low Lectin FoodFrame can be beneficial for anyone, especially those with inflammation, as it improves digestion and gut issues like bloating, heartburn, and acid reflux. It supports anyone with blood sugar issues, making it a good choice for those who prefer not to go on the Keto or Paleo FoodFrames. It is also an effective way to see weight loss, a decrease in joint pain, improved mood, and better sleep. It can improve leaky gut, IBS, and systemic inflammation as well.

SIDEBAR – Tamara's Story

Tamara was bright and well-educated and like most people had never been to a nutritionist, placing faith in her doctors. She had been diagnosed with Common Variable Immune Deficiency (CVID), a disorder that impairs the immune system. People with CVID are highly susceptible to infection from foreign invaders such as bacteria, or, more rarely, viruses; they often develop recurrent infections, particularly in the lungs, sinuses, and ears. Not surprisingly, Tamara had a chronic sinus infection which she treated with antibiotics and steroids for the better part of a year. In addition, she had asthma, regular headaches, and migraines; diarrhea several times a week for years; anxiety; and full body aches daily.

This was a long list of symptoms, and following my detox, I immediately put her on a Low Lectin FoodFrame. Removing certain foods quelled the inflammation in her gut and stopped the diarrhea. She also tested positive for the gene mutation MTHFR so once we addressed that with the proper B vitamin, her panic attacks were eliminated entirely. Doing the water aerobics she loved helped lower her anxiety levels, too.

Tamara was initially reluctant to give up the nightshades and other foods that were high in lectins, but once she did, she was rewarded handsomely. Her asthma and sinus infections occurred less frequently. I suggested she also remove all alcohol, gluten, and dairy from her diet. When Tamara is compliant, she sees 100 % results. When she goes out of the box, she immediately experiences diarrhea and body aches… and goes right back to the Low Lectin FoodFrame!

WHO SHOULD AVOID THIS DIET

There really isn't anyone who wouldn't benefit from this diet, but it is certainly challenging for vegetarians as their main source of protein is usually legumes and grains. Also, for those who love lectin-rich foods--especially tomatoes, potatoes, grains, and legumes--the restrictions can be challenging. As it is for those who have to travel a lot and have little control over where they'll be eating.

LOW LECTIN FOODS TO ENJOY

Meat

*Includes broth and collagen

Cattle (beef, veal), deer (venison), goat, hare, pig (pork), rabbit, sheep (lamb, mutton), wild game (buffalo/bison, boar, elk)

Poultry

Includes broth and collagen

Chicken, duck, goose, grouse, guinea hen, ostrich, pheasant, quail, turkey

Fish

Includes broth and collagen

Anchovy, arctic char, bass, bonito, carp, catfish, cod, eel, gar, haddock, hake, halibut, herring, mackerel, mahi-mahi, marlin, monkfish, perch, pollock, salmon, sardine, snapper, sole, swordfish, tilapia, trout, tuna (ahi, yellowfin), turbot, walleye

Shellfish

Includes broth and collagen

Clams, crab, crawfish, lobster, mussels, octopus, oysters, scallops, shrimp, squid

Eggs

Chicken, duck, goose, quail, including fish eggs/caviar

Plant Protein

Hemp tofu, tempeh

Dairy

A2 milk, 1 oz cheese or 4 oz yogurt per day; buffalo mozzarella, coconut yogurt, organic cream cheese, goat cheese, goat and sheep kefir, organic heavy cream, high fat cheeses (brie), sheep cheese, organic sour cream

Leafy Vegetables

Unlimited

Arugula, beet greens, Bok choy, broccoli rabe, Brussels sprouts, cabbage, carrot tops, celery, chicory, collard greens, cress, dandelion greens, endive, kale - all varieties, lettuce - all varieties, mustard greens, Napa cabbage, purslane, radicchio, sorrel, spinach, Swiss chard, tatsoi, turnip greens, watercress

Non-starchy Vegetables

Artichoke, asparagus, broccoli, cauliflower, celery, fennel, rhubarb, squash blossoms

Allium-family Vegetables

Chive, garlic, leek, onion, scallion, shallot, wild leek

Roots, Tubers, and Bulb Vegetables

Arrowroot, bamboo shoot, beet, burdock, carrot, cassava, celeriac, daikon, ginger, horseradish and root, Jerusalem artichoke, jicama, kohlrabi, lotus root, parsnip, radish, rutabaga, sweet potato, taro, turnip, wasabi, water chestnut, yam, yam noodles

Sea Vegetables

Arame, dulse, hijiki, kombu, nori, wakame

Vegetable-like Fruits

Avocado, okra, olives

Berries

0-1 serving daily, only in season

Blackberry, blueberry, raspberry, strawberry

Citrus-family Fruits

Lemon, lime and kiwi

Edible Fungi/Mushrooms

Chanterelle, cremini, morel, oyster, porcini, portobello, shiitake, truffle

Animal Fats

Bacon fat, butter (grass-fed or European), ghee, lard, leaf lard (fat from pig), pan drippings, poultry fat, schmaltz (chicken or goose fat), strutto (clarified pork fat), tallow (from beef, lamb, or mutton)

Plant Fats

Algae oil, avocado oil (cold-pressed), coconut oil, cod liver oil, extra-virgin olive oil (cold-pressed), macadamia oil, MCT oil, perilla oil, red palm shortening, rice bran, sesame oil, walnut oil,

Nuts/Nut Butters and Nut Oils

½ cup daily

Almonds, Brazil nuts, chestnuts, hazelnuts, macadamia, pecans, pine nuts, pistachios, walnuts

Seeds and Seed Oils

Flax seeds, hemp seeds, poppy seeds, psyllium, sesame seeds

Probiotic Foods

Fermented meat or fish, kombucha (in moderation), kvass, lacto-fermented fruits and vegetables, non-dairy kefir, sauerkraut

Herbs and Spices

Allspice, anise, annatto, basil leaf, bay leaf, black caraway, cardamom, celery seed, chamomile, Chinese five-spice powder, chervil, chives, cilantro, coriander, cinnamon, cloves, cumin, curry powder, dill, fennel seed, fennel leaf, fenugreek, garlic, ginger, garam masala, juniper, kaffir lime leaf, lavender, lemongrass, mace, marjoram leaf, mustard, nutmeg, onion powder, oregano leaf, parsley, pepper, peppermint, poppy, rosemary, saffron, sage, savory leaf, sea or Himalayan salt, spearmint, tarragon, thyme, turmeric, vanilla

Flours

Almond, arrowroot, cassava, chestnut, coconut, hazelnut, sesame, grape seed, green banana, sweet potato, tapioca, Tiger nut

Flavorings

Watch for added ingredients

Anchovy paste, apple cider vinegar, balsamic vinegar, capers, carob powder, coconut aminos (a soy sauce substitute), coconut concentrate, coconut milk, coconut water vinegar, fish sauce, fruit and vegetable juice (in moderation), organic chutneys and jams (in moderation), red wine vinegar, truffle oil (made with olive oil), white wine vinegar

Desserts

Coconut milk ice cream made with sugar alcohols, dark chocolate (72% +)

Sweeteners

In moderation

Allulose, erythritol, inulin, stevia, monk fruit (Luo Han Guo), and monk fruit flavored maple syrup, xylitol, yacon

Alcohol

Aged spirits (1 oz daily), champagne (maximum 1 6-oz glass daily), red wine (max 1 6-oz glass daily),

Beverages

Water (club, mineral, reverse osmosis, seltzer, soda, sparkling [without natural flavors, sweeteners, or additives], spring); almond milk (unsweetened), coconut milk, coconut water (in moderation), green or black tea (in moderation), green juices (freshly squeezed, no fruit), hemp milk (unsweetened), herbal teas, yerba mate (in moderation)

Grain in Moderation

Millet

LOW LECTIN FOODS TO AVOID

Grains and Grain-Like Foods

Amaranth, barley, buckwheat, bulgur, corn, farro, oats/oatmeal, quinoa, rice, rye, sorghum, spelt, teff, wheat (all varieties, including einkorn and semolina), wheat kamut, whole grains, wild rice

Tropical fruits

Acerola, banana, chayote, cherimoya, coconut, date, dragon fruit, durian, fig, guava, jackfruit, kiwi, loquat, lychee, mango, mangosteen, papaya, passion fruit, pawpaw, persimmon, pineapple, plantain, pomegranate, star fruit, tamarind

Dairy

Buttermilk, butter, casein protein powders, cheeses (American, cottage, low-fat, ricotta), creams (low-fat), kefir (cow's milk), yogurt (frozen or Greek)

Legumes

Adzuki beans, black beans, black-eyed peas, butter beans, calico beans, cannellini beans, chickpeas (garbanzo beans), fava beans (broad beans), great northern beans, green beans, Italian beans, kidney beans, lentils, lima beans, mung beans, navy beans, peanuts, peas, pinto beans, runner beans, soybeans (including edamame, tofu, tempeh, other soy products, and soy isolates, such as soy lecithin), split peas

Nightshades or Spices Derived from Nightshades

Ashwagandha, capsicums/peppers, chili pepper flakes, chili powder, curry, cayenne pepper, paprika, pepinos, peppers (bell, chipotle, hot, red, and sweet), and pimentos; cape gooseberries, eggplant, goji berries (wolfberries), potatoes (sweet potatoes and yams are not nightshades and are okay), sweet plantains, tomatoes (all varieties unless peeled and deseeded)

Rosaceae-family Fruits

Apple, apricot, cherry, nectarine, peach, pear, plum, quince, rosehip

Melons

Cantaloupe, honeydew, horned melon, melon pear, Persian melon, watermelon, winter melon

Citrus-family Fruits

Clementine, grapefruit, kumquat, orange, pomelo, tangelo, tangerine, yuzu

Vegetable-like Fruits

Bitter melon, chayote, cucumber, plantain, pumpkin, squashes (all), winter melon, zucchini (unless peeled and deseeded)

Nuts/Nut Butters and Nut Oils

Cashews, peanuts

Seeds and Seed Oils

Chia seeds, pumpkin seeds, sunflower seeds

Seasonings and Condiments

Chili pepper flakes, ketchup, mayonnaise, soy sauce, steak sauces

Processed Vegetable Oils

Canola oil (rapeseed oil), corn oil, cottonseed oil, grapeseed oil, palm kernel oil, peanut oil, safflower oil, soybean oil, sunflower oil

*In moderation

Processed Food Chemicals and Ingredients

Acrylamides, artificial food color, autolyzed protein, brominated vegetable oil, emulsifiers (carrageenan, soy lecithin), hydrolyzed vegetable protein, monosodium glutamate, nitrates or nitrites (naturally occurring are okay), olestra, phosphoric acid, propylene glycol, textured vegetable protein, trans fats (partially hydrogenated vegetable oil, hydrogenated oil), yeast extract

Sugars

Agave, agave nectar, barley malt, barley malt syrup, beet sugar, brown rice syrup, brown sugar, cane crystals, cane juice, cane sugar, raw cane sugar, evaporated cane juice, and dehydrated cane juice, caramel, coconut sugar, coconut syrup, corn sweetener, corn syrup and corn syrup solids, crystalline fructose, date sugar, demerara sugar, dextrin, dextrose, fructose, high-fructose corn syrup, fruit juice, fruit juice concentrate, glucose, glucose solids, golden syrup, raw honey, invert sugar, jaggery, lactose, lucuma, malt syrup, maltodextrin, maltose, maple sugar, maple syrup, molasses, muscovado sugar, palm sugar, raw sugar, refined sugar, rice bran syrup, rice syrup, saccharose, sorghum syrup, sucanat, sucrose, syrup, treacle, turbinado sugar

Sugar Alcohols

Naturally occurring sugar alcohols found in whole foods like fruit are okay

Mannitol, sorbitol

Non-nutritive Sweeteners

Acesulfame potassium, aspartame (Sweet 'n Low, Equal), neotame, saccharin, stevia, sucralose (Splenda)

Nuts and Nut Oils

Peanuts, peanut oil

Alcohol

All beer, liquor, wine, or any other form of alcoholic beverages are technically not permitted (small amounts in kombucha are okay). Some choose to have alcohol in moderation; distilled liquors like vodka, tequila, or gin are the best choices with sparkling water and lemon or lime

Beverages

Any drinks containing artificial coloring, flavors, sweeteners, or preservatives; coffee (decaf and caffeinated), cow milk, electrolyte drinks, energy drinks, fruit juices, kefir (dairy-based), rice milk, sodas (diet and regular), soymilk, sports drinks

LIFE AFTER THE LOW LECTIN FOODFRAME

The Low Lectin FoodFrame is an eating lifestyle so it can be followed for a lifetime. If you go out of the low lectin box, make sure to pop right back in as soon as you can. It is essentially a hybrid between Paleo and AIP as there is a lot of crossover with them both. Most people with joint pain and inflammation will feel the effects when eating foods not permitted, which I love as this is such a tangible sign that your body is telling you what it wants. Best to listen to it!

Again, I always encourage people to choose the FoodFrame that suits their health status, lifestyle, and preferences. Keep trying what works best for you until you find the perfect FoodFrame!

LOW LECTIN - RECIPES

Lemon Meringue Shake

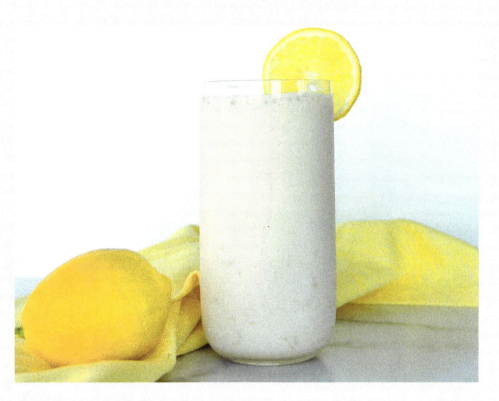

Ingredients:

½ cup lemon juice (juice of 2 lemons)
⅔ cup coconut milk or unsweetened almond milk
1 scoop RGN Collagen Protein, vanilla
½ teaspoon monk fruit, stevia or allulose

1-2 pinches sea salt
1 teaspoon vanilla extract
1 cup lemon extract
1 tablespoon coconut cream

Instructions:

Place all ingredients in a blender and blend until smooth.

Serves 1

Sweet Potato Toast

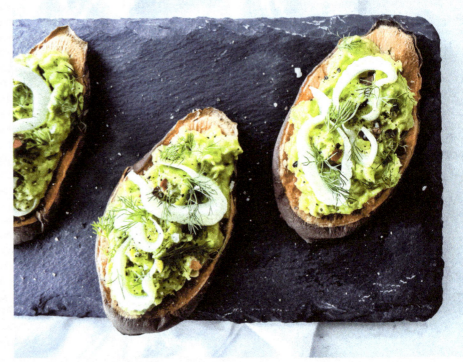

Ingredients:

½ sweet potato, large

For Mashed Avocado:
1 ripe avocado
Sea salt to taste

For Sautéed Spinach:
½ tablespoon ghee or coconut oil
1-2 garlic cloves, minced
2-4 handfuls of organic spinach
Sea salt to taste

For Sautéed Mushrooms:
½ tablespoon ghee or coconut oil
1-2 cups sliced mushrooms of your choice
1 teaspoon fresh rosemary, chopped
Sea salt to taste

Instructions:

1. Preheat oven or toaster oven at 375 degrees.
2. Wash the sweet potato while leaving skin on. Slice lengthwise into ¼-inch thick slices.
3. Bake slices in oven or toaster oven for 20-25 minutes or until soft and starting to brown. Top with your choice of toppings.

Toppings Instructions:

Mashed Avocado:
Remove skin and pit from avocado and mash until desired consistency. Add sea salt to taste.

Sauteed Spinach:
Melt ghee or coconut oil in pan on medium heat. Add spinach and stir until the leaves start to wilt. Add garlic and sea salt to taste.

Sauteed Mushrooms:
Melt ghee or coconut oil in pan on medium heat. Add mushrooms and rosemary and stir until mushrooms are slightly wilted. Add sea salt to taste.

Serves 2-4

Mediterranean Chicken

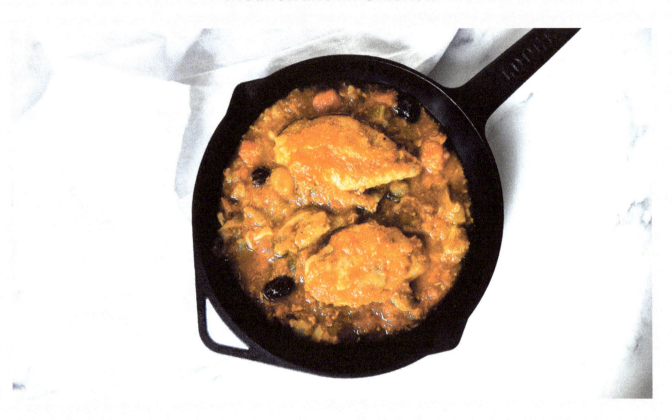

🍴 Ingredients:

1 tablespoon avocado or coconut oil
6 pastured boneless chicken breasts
4 large orange carrots, peeled and trimmed
3 cups chicken broth (I use Bonafide Provisions)
1 cup pearl onions, fresh or frozen
12 oz. artichoke hearts, quartered or halved

2 cups cremini mushrooms, quartered
1 tablespoon fresh rosemary, chopped
1 tablespoon fresh oregano, chopped
Sea salt and pepper to taste
1 large handful organic spinach
1 cup Kalamata olives, pitted and halved lengthwise

Instructions:

1. Place oil and chicken in a large soup pot or large saucepan and cook on medium heat.
2. Add bone broth along with the onions, artichokes, and mushrooms. Stir, turn chicken, then cover.
3. While the chicken and vegetables are cooking, chop the carrots into pieces and steam for 10 minutes until they are completely soft. Strain and puree in a food processor or high-speed blender.
4. Add the carrot puree along with the rosemary, oregano, sea salt, and pepper to the soup pot. Cook for 10-15 minutes.
5. Add spinach and olives. Cover and gently cook for another 5 minutes.

If you want it saucier, add a bit of bone broth or water.

Optional: Serve over cauliflower rice

Serves 6

Risa Groux, CN

Turmeric Cauliflower Rice

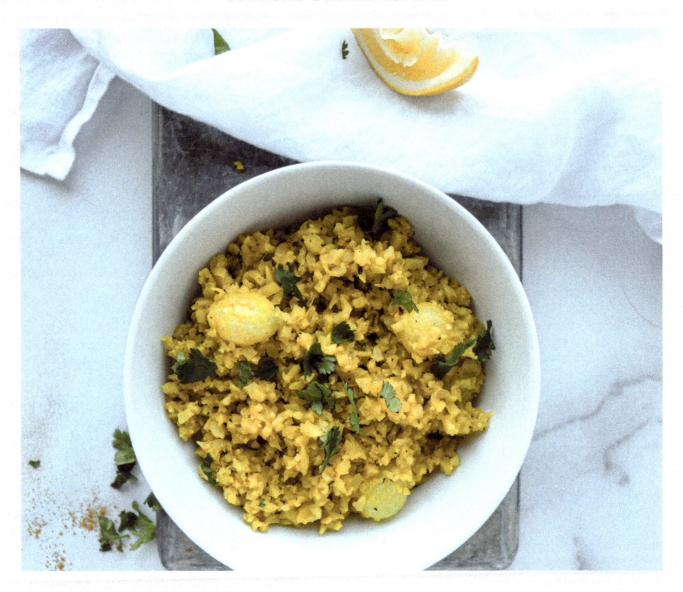

Ingredients:

1 tablespoon coconut or avocado oil
½ yellow or white onion, chopped
2-3 garlic cloves, minced
2 12 oz. bags riced cauliflower

1 tablespoon ground turmeric
½ tablespoon curry powder
1 tablespoon ghee
Sea salt and pepper to taste

Instructions:

1. In a large skillet on medium heat, melt coconut oil or heat avocado oil. Add garlic and onions. Stir until onions are translucent, approximately 3-5 minutes.
2. Add the cauliflower rice, turmeric and curry. Mix until well combined.
3. Add ghee, sea salt, and pepper to taste. Cook for approximately 5-7 more minutes.

Serve with an animal protein or roasted vegetables.

Serves 4-6

Creamy Mushroom Soup

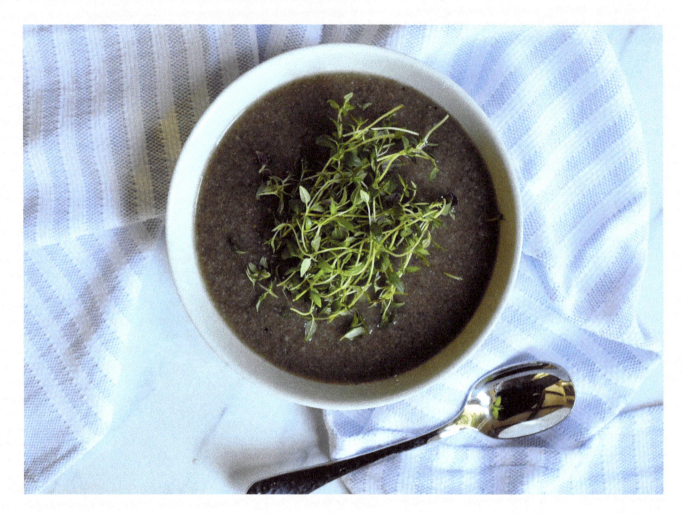

🍴 Ingredients:

1-2 tablespoons ghee
3 garlic cloves, minced
1 medium white or yellow onion, chopped
10 oz cremini mushrooms, sliced
10 oz white mushrooms, sliced

3-5 oz shiitake mushrooms, sliced
4-6 cups bone broth
1 teaspoon fresh or dried thyme
Sea salt and pepper to taste

Instructions:

1. In a soup pan on medium heat, melt ghee and add garlic, onion, mushrooms, and stir occasionally until all ingredients are soft.
2. Add bone broth and heat until cooked through, approximately 10 minutes.
3. Using a hand or regular blender, blend the soup until smooth.
4. Add thyme, sea salt and pepper.

Optional: For a cream soup add ½ cup coconut milk.

Garnish with sautéed mushrooms and/or Italian parsley.

Serves 6-8

Lemon Cookies

🍴 Ingredients:

½ cup coconut oil, melted
⅔ cup monk fruit maple syrup
2 tablespoons lemon zest
3 teaspoons lemon extract
2-⅔ cups blanched almond flour
4 tablespoons coconut flour
1 teaspoon baking soda
¼ teaspoon sea salt

🍴 Instructions:

Preheat the oven to 350 degrees and line two baking sheets with parchment paper.

1. In a large bowl, mix the coconut oil, maple syrup, lemon zest, and lemon extract. Add the almond flour, coconut flour, baking soda and sea salt. If the dough is a bit wet, do *not* add any additional flour simply place in the refrigerator for up to 30 minutes to firm it up.
2. Roll dough into balls and place 3-inches apart on baking sheet. Slightly flatten the cookie dough balls with the palm of your hand. Bake for 12-15 minutes or until the cookies have lightly browned on the bottom and sides. The cookies may crack a little on the edges.

Makes 10-12 cookies

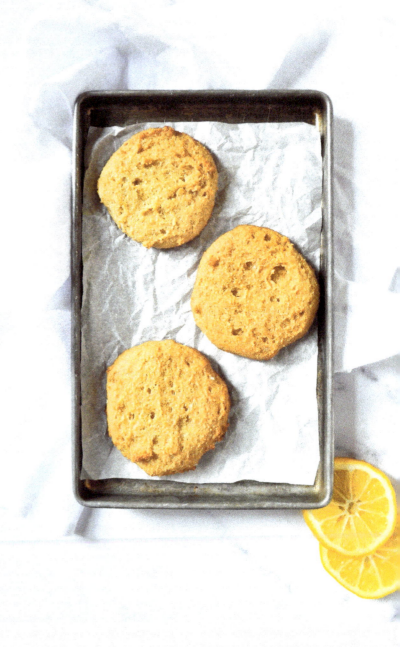

CHAPTER 9

THE LOW FODMAP FOODFRAME

Irritable Bowel Syndrome (IBS) and Irritable Bowel Disease (IBD) are essentially inflammation of the bowel. Both are chronic conditions with the potential of causing abdominal pain, cramping, constipation, and often diarrhea with bowel movement urgency. IBS is described as inflammation in the digestive tract, typically the lower end of the large intestines and colon. IBD is a term used to describe a cluster of digestive disorders such as Crohn's disease, ulcerative colitis, and diverticulitis. IBD is caused by inflammation in the bowel and the symptoms can be more severe than IBS, such as blood in the stool, black and tarry stools, and loss of appetite.

IBS and IBD are both typically blanket diagnoses provided when there is general intestinal inflammation and no specific conclusion such as Crohn's disease, ulcerative colitis, or diverticulitis. If IBS goes untreated, you are susceptible to dehydration as well as mineral and nutrient deficiency which all lead to chronic disease.

Another extremely common and drastically undiagnosed condition is called SIBO, short for Small Intestinal Bacteria Overgrowth. We all house bacteria in our large intestine, and SIBO can happen when bacteria accidently park themselves in the small intestines, where it starts to ferment sugars and fibers. This leads to abdominal distress--excessive gas, chronic bloating, abdominal pain and cramping, nausea, constipation or diarrhea, and/or weight loss. If SIBO goes untreated for an extended period of time, additional health concerns such as malnutrition due to malabsorption, megaloblastic anemia, peripheral neuropathy, night blindness, and even osteoporosis can occur.

Low FODMAP is an elimination FoodFrame which helps alleviate the symptoms of IBS, IBD, and SIBO naturally. Certain foods can directly impact the cascade of inflammation, so when you stop eating them, your gut can begin to heal.

FODMAP is an acronym for each food category that perpetuates the overgrowth and inflammation in the intestinal lining. These categories are:

- **F**ermentable
- **O**ligosaccharides - Fructans: wheat, garlic, onions, inulin, artichokes; and galacto-oligosaccharides: legumes, lentils, garbanzo beans
- **D**isaccharides – Lactose-containing foods: all forms of milk, yogurt, ice cream, soft cheeses that are not aged
- **M**onosaccharides - Fructose foods: honey, agave, apples, pears, mangoes, watermelon, and high fructose corn syrup
And
- **P**olyols - Sugar alcohols and fructose: erythritol, sorbitol, mannitol; avocados, apples, cherries, nectarines, prunes, and mushrooms.

TESTING FOR GUT INFLAMMATION

Testing for these diagnoses can be a bit challenging. There are no concrete tests that result in a positive diagnosis, but rather a series of tests for inflammation that will lead to a conclusive diagnosis.

Testing for IBS and IBD

Many physicians will diagnose IBS based on symptoms, family history, and a physical exam. From my experience, a stool test is the most accurate for IBS. An inflammation marker called Calprotectin is most often elevated, indicating the level of inflammation in the intestinal tract to confirm IBS. If significantly elevated and out of lab range, this marker will usually indicate some form of IBS either present or in the making. We typically see this marker with numerous symptoms, but it can also exist without significant symptoms.

Testing for IBD is usually done through blood tests, x-rays, and colonoscopy. Always check with your physician or gastroenterologist.

Testing for SIBO

Testing for SIBO is a bit tricky. Blood tests often give both false positives and false negatives, so I don't recommend them. Breath tests are commonly used by physicians in their office or a kit can be sent to the patient's home. To prepare for the test, you need to eat a limited diet 1-2 days prior, then drink a prescribed sugar-containing liquid, followed by breathing into several tubes every 20 minutes for three hours to measure the methane and hydrogen amounts produced by your body. This test is commonly used, but often creates a substantial number of false negatives. Stool tests are best but not a perfect solution either. Since not all stool tests are created equal, be sure to get one that includes testing for the bacteria Methanobacteriacai and Bacillus species. Methanobacteriacai is an opportunistic intestinal bacterium that produces methane gas, which causes bloating and is a common symptom with SIBO. That along with a flagged or out-of-range Bacillus species (spp), another opportunistic bacterium, can be very conclusive if SIBO symptoms are present as well.

The unscientific test that anyone can do at home (and is much more enjoyable!) is to eat approximately 15-25 plantain chips on an empty stomach. If you bloat after fifteen to thirty minutes, it is highly likely SIBO exists. Plantains contain resistant starches, so they are very reactive and not helpful for anyone with IBS or SIBO.

SIDEBAR - Common SIBO Symptom

- Abdominal Pain
- Asthma
- Belching
- Bloating
- Constipation
- Depression
- Diarrhea
- Fatigue
- Gas
- Nausea and vomiting
- Skin rashes; acne, eczema, rosacea
- Weight loss

Treating SIBO

SIBO can be treated effectively with three very different approaches. Since SIBO has a high incidence of recurrence, everyone will have a different experience with what works and how long to adhere to the protocol. Upon recurrence, an eating plan and supplements can usually reverse the symptoms. In tough cases, I have seen clients do all three protocols concurrently or back-to-back with great success.

1. **Antibiotics**. An antibiotic called Xifaxan (also known as Rifaximin) can eradicate several strains of the bacteria. This is often prescribed for 10-21 days and doesn't destroy as much of the good bacteria as other antibiotics do. Most people I know start here and then dive into protocol #2.
2. **Low FODMAP Diet**. The second method is the Low FODMAP diet paired with a specific supplement protocol. The supplements are composed of herbal antibiotics and anti-fungals geared to eradicate the bacteria with minimal gut microbiome destruction and are taken for several consecutive weeks depending on the severity and overall gut health. In addition, I recommend a probiotic either during the protocol or after, but always making sure the probiotic does not contain a prebiotic as that will feed the bacteria you are trying to eliminate. I use this in my office with a high degree of success--but compliance is key.
3. **The Elemental Diet**. This is a liquid-only protocol with suggested use of 14-28 days. The nutrients are in an assimilated form so your body can absorb them with minimal disruption to the gut, with the intent to support healing and assist in the killing of bacteria in the small intestine. I have seen this to be effective, but usually not as a stand-alone treatment. Drinking liquids throughout the day with no food to eat can be quite challenging, so it's not for everyone. It's more typically a last resort for very tough SIBO cases.

WHO LOW FODMAP IS BEST FOR

If you have been diagnosed with IBS; IBD conditions such as Crohn's disease, colitis (all forms), diverticulitis; or SIBO, this diet is for you. Even if you haven't had formal testing yet suspect you have one of these conditions as you regularly experience some or many of the symptoms, enjoying a Low FODMAP diet could improve how well you feel. The diet is designed to eliminate or severely minimize foods that cause bloating or gas, so anyone with those symptoms should experience immediate relief.

There are a few stages to this diet; the first is most restrictive, especially when it comes to portion size, which is key. Someone can feel great with one-quarter cup of broccoli but not an ounce more. I cannot emphasize this enough--portion size is imperative here for success! It is critical to listen to your body to see what it can tolerate.

Once you become less symptomatic, you can advance to the next stage. This is intended to alleviate discomfort and begin healing your intestines. Out of all the diets, this one is very dependent on the individual. What works for someone may not work for you--and the only way to know is by trying.

SIDEBAR – Zach's Story

When Zach was in college, he enjoyed social time at his fraternity. This involved a certain amount of drinking and eating a lot of junk food. He began noticing sensitivities to certain foods, extensive daily bloating, and bad breath. He'd received a confirmed diagnosis of SIBO from his doctor after a breath test and was prescribed a round of Rifaximin for 10 days. This made Zach feel better, but all his symptoms returned once he completed the protocol. I immediately ordered a stool test and suggested the Low FODMAP FoodFrame to prevent bloating and gave him natural supplements that would kill the bacteria that had lodged in his small intestine. He was willing to curtail his drinking with friends until he saw results. I also recommended an app he could use when he was food shopping or out with friends and gave him lots of recipe options from my website. Almost immediately the bloating went away, and while working to restore the integrity of his intestinal lining, his bad breath disappeared as well.

Because SIBO is highly reoccurring, Zach knows if he gets off-track it will come back, so he stays on a Low FODMAP FoodFrame for the most part and dials it up at the onset of any symptoms. He travels extensively for work but has learned how to eat to maximize his health.

WHO SHOULD AVOID THE LOW FODMAP FOODFRAME

Following a Low FODMAP FoodFrame wouldn't hurt anyone, but it is not recommended for those who do not experience any bloating or digestive issues. This diet is limiting and can be hard to maintain, especially when dining out—which makes it difficult for those who travel a lot, have many business meetings, or family gatherings over meals. The largest obstacle while at restaurants tend to be onions and garlic, as they're commonly used in many of the most common foods for all ethnicities.

HOW LOW FODMAP WORKS

The theory behind the Low FODMAP FoodFrame is to minimize or prevent short-chain carbohydrate foods that draw water into the digestive tract, which can lead to excessive gas, bloating, diarrhea, or constipation. Foods that are high in FODMAPS feed the bacteria, which ferments the sugars and fibers, causing abdominal distress and chronic discomfort, while perpetuating SIBO.

Monash University in Melbourne Australia was the first to formulate the Low FODMAP diet. Since then, practitioners may have their own slightly altered version of it, so it is common to see a variety of iterations due to more research being released. Originally, bananas were considered safe or Low FODMAP if sticking to a half-cup or half a banana. Recent research has shown that riper bananas are higher in FODMAPS, so they're now suggesting restricting bananas; you would probably be fine, however, with the original dose but with a greener banana. In addition, zucchini has now been discovered to be on the higher side versus yellow summer squash. While Monash continues to research FODMAPS, the lists will continue to evolve, but I always recommend watching portion size and seeing how your body reacts. You can always find up-to-date information on the Monash University FODMAP Diet App.

This diet is also tricky as many people can tolerate small amounts of high FODMAP foods, so it's not a one-size-fits-all program. It is recommended to be followed to the letter for exactly four weeks, and then start to reintroduce in small amounts one specific category of foods at a time. Quantity is a critical factor during the elimination phase, so initially adhering to these restrictions will have the best results.

LOW FODMAP FOODS TO ENJOY

NOTE: Because portion control is so individual, this list contains foods you can enjoy and those you should avoid, but not the quantities. Every person reacts differently to these foods, so only you can be the judge of what is best for your body.

Protein

Beef, chicken, eggs (including caviar), fish, pork (including bacon without HFCS), RGN collagen protein powder, tofu

Dairy

Butter, dry curd and lactose-free cottage cheese, lactose free cow milk, lactose-free cream cheese, lactose-free yogurt, labneh, ghee, yogurt (coconut, goat milk, or lactose-free)

Vegetables and Leafy Greens

Arugula, bamboo shoots, beets (cooked or pickled) 1 oz, Bok choy, beets (pickled), bell peppers, broccoli,

Brussels sprouts (2), butternut squash (¼ cup serving), cabbage, carrots, celery root/celeriac, chard, chives, collard greens, cucumber, eggplant, endive, fennel bulb and stalk, green beans, ginger root, kabocha squash, kale, lettuce, nori seaweed, olives, parsnip, patty pan squash, peas, peppers (bell, sweet, chili), sweet potato (½ cup serving), whole or pureed pumpkin (canned, ¼ cup serving), radish, rutabaga, scallions and leeks (green part only), spaghetti squash, spinach, Swiss chard, summer squash, tomatoes (all varieties), turnip, watercress, zucchini

Fruit

*Limit to one-quarter cup serving per meal or otherwise noted

Banana (small, firm, ⅓ max), blueberries, boysenberry, cantaloupe, clementine, coconut (¼ cup fresh, or dried), dried current (1 tbsp), dragon fruit, dried cranberries (1 tbsp), grapes, guava, honeydew, kiwi, longan, lemon, lime, orange, papaya, passion fruit, pineapple, pomegranate (½ small), prickly pear, raisins, rambutan, raspberries, rhubarb, star fruit, strawberries, tangelo, tangerine

Grains and Grain-Like Foods

*Note: Gluten is not a FODMAP, but many gluten-free products tend to be low in FODMAPs.

Gluten-free bread, gluten-free pasta, millet, oats, polenta, quinoa, quinoa flakes, rice, rice cakes, slow-leavened sourdough wheat or spelt bread, soba noodles, tortillas (corn only)

Nuts and Seeds

*Limit to 15 nuts or fewer per day/2-6 teaspoons of seeds per day

Almonds, brazil nuts, coconut, chestnuts, hazelnuts, macadamias, peanuts, pecans, pine nuts, poppy seeds, pumpkin seeds, sesame seeds, sunflower seeds, walnuts

Oils

Bacon fat, butter, coconut oil, cod liver/fish oil, duck fat, garlic infused oil, ghee, lard, and tallow, MCT oil, macadamia oil, olive oil, palm oil, vegetable oils (canola, flax, grape seed, hemp, pumpkin seed, sesame oil, sunflower oil, walnut oil

Legumes

Lentils (½ cup, canned, drained, and rinsed), lima, tempeh (plain)

Herbs

Basil, cilantro, coriander, lemongrass, mint, mustard greens, rosemary, parsley, sage, tarragon, thyme

Sweeteners

Brown sugar, cocoa powder, dark chocolate, honey, monk fruit, palm sugar, raw sugar, stevia, vanilla, white sugar

Desserts

Rice milk and other lactose-free ice cream, sorbet from acceptable fruits

Beverages

All servings of juice should be 4 oz or less

Apple and raspberry cordial, canned coconut milk (full fat and light), coffee (1 cup per day, use non-dairy milk or creamers, or a splash of lactose-free cow's milk), fruit juice not from concentrate, milk (lactose-free cow's milk [whole, 2%, 1%, or fat-free]; unsweetened almond, hemp, or rice milk), juice from low FODMAP fruits, tea flavored with ginger and cinnamon (1-2 cups per day of black tea, ginger, green, rooibos, buchu, hibiscus, honeybush, chai tea [made weak], dandelion tea [made weak]); water (carbonated, infused, or spring)

Alcohol

Occasional drinking only

Bourbon, gin, vodka, whiskey, scotch, wine

Bars

RGN Collagen Paleo Bar

LOW FODMAP FOODS TO AVOID

Protein

Processed meats with additives, carrageenan, sugar, high fructose corn syrup

Vegetables

Artichokes (Jerusalem, globe, pickled in oil), asparagus (1 spear), beansprouts, beetroot, bitter melon, broccoli, Brussels sprouts, cabbage, savoy, cauliflower, chicory leaves, corn kernels, garlic (including garlic powder), leeks (only leaves are low), dried lotus root, dried mushroom - all except oyster mushrooms are permitted, okra, onions (pickled and onion powder), peas - all varieties, scallion, seaweed, spring onion bulbs (only use green tips), shallots, starch powder (arrowroot, corn, potato, rice, tapioca) taro, turnip, water chestnuts, yam, yucca

Legumes

* ¼ cup cooked unless ½ cup is noted

Baked beans, black beans (¼ cup boiled, canned is okay), black-eyed peas, borlotti beans, broad beans, butter beans, chickpeas (garbanzo beans), fava, haricot beans, kidney beans, lentils (¼ cup red or green, boiled is permitted; ½ cup canned lentils),

¼ cup canned chickpeas are permitted if they are drained from the can and rinsed before consuming, navy beans, and boiled red kidney beans, soya beans, boiled, soybeans, split peas

Nuts and Seeds

Cashews, chia seeds, seed flours, pistachios

Fruit

Apples (fresh or dried), applesauce, apricots (fresh, dried, canned), Asian pears, avocado, banana (ripe, ⅓ maximum is permitted), blackberries, boysenberries, cherries, currants (1 tablespoon or less), dates, figs (fresh or dried), goji berries (dried, 1 tablespoon or less), grapefruit, guava (preferably unripe but ripe is permitted), jackfruit (freeze-dried), lychee, mango (fresh or dried), nectarines, peaches (all), pears (dried or ripe), persimmon, pineapple (dried only), plum (black diamond), prunes, raisins (1 tablespoon or less), watermelon

Dairy

All dairy milk (A2, evaporated, sweetened, condensed, regular, full cream, cow/goat, skim and reduced fat, condensed milk, cottage cheese, cream, cream cheese, soft cheeses (2 tablespoons or less is permitted), chéve, cream, crème fraiche, custard, ice cream, feta, goat, milk powder (milk solids), mozzarella, parmesan, pecorino, pudding made from milk (read labels on lactose-free and vegan puddings), ricotta, Swiss, sour cream

Yogurt

Cow/sheep's milk, flavored, kefir, low-fat, regular

Non-Dairy Milk

Coconut milk made with inulin, oat milk (½ cup or less), soymilk (made from soy protein is permitted in small quantities)

Meat Additives

Meats containing onion, garlic, onion or garlic powders; breadcrumbs, dehydrated powders, dried fruits; meats prepared with gravy, marinades, or sauces

Vegetarian Substitutes

Falafel, lentil burger, silken tofu (not firm), soy protein, (textured, TVP)

Grains and Baking

Avoid if they contain wheat, rye, or barley

Amaranth, barley, bread, breadcrumbs, bulgur, cakes, chickpea flour (in small amounts is permitted), cookies, couscous, crackers, croissants, durum, lentil flour (in small amounts is permitted), muffins, multigrain flour, pastries, pea flour (in small amounts is permitted), pizza, rye, semolina, sourdough, soy flour (in small amounts is permitted), triticale, wheat bran, wheat flour, wheat germ

Pasta/Cereal

Avoid wheat-based

Gnocchi, muesli, multi-grain breakfast cereal, noodles, pasta

Snacks: Bars and Cookies

All: Cereal bars, cookies, energy bars, fruit and nut bars, fruit-filled cookies, granola bars, muesli-based bars made with fruit, oatmeal bars, peanut butter bars, rye crispbread

Oils

Soybean oil

Seasonings

Chicory root, gums, soy sauce, tamari, onion and garlic powder, balsamic vinegar. Watch for onion and garlic-based sauces and marinades that are high FODMAPS

Additives

Carrageenan, thickeners

Condiments and Sauces

Brand-made relishes, chutneys, dressings, gravies, hummus, oil-based sauces and condiments, pasta sauces, stock (beef, chicken, or vegetable), tzatziki dip, and beef, chicken and vegetable, bouillon cubes

Sweeteners

Agave nectar and syrup, all berry jams and jellies (made with high fructose corn syrup, apple juice, pear juice, or other high-FODMAPs), barley malt syrup, brown rice syrup, cane sugar, cocoa/chocolate unsweetened, coconut sugar, fructose, fruit juice concentrate (any), high fructose corn syrup, maple syrup, molasses, sugar (sucrose), sucralose

Sugar Alcohols

Avoid label warnings that say: "Excess consumption may have a laxative effect"

Erythritol, isomalt, lactitol, maltitol, mannitol, polydextrose (a combination of dextrose, a corn sugar, and sorbitol), sorbitol, xylitol

Beverages

Coconut milk with thickeners, fruit juice concentrates and those from high FODMAP fruits, energy drinks, soda, sports drinks, tea (chicory root, licorice, pau d'arco)

Coffee and Tea

Carob powder (for drinking), chamomile tea, chicory-based coffee, coconut water (8 oz or less is permitted), espresso, decaf or regular (with cow milk or soymilk), fennel tea, instant decaf or regular coffee (with cow milk or soymilk), oolong tea

Alcohol

Beer, brandy, hard cider, liqueurs/cordials, rum, sherry, tequila, fortified/dessert wine, sweet wine, sparkling wine, port

LIFE AFTER LOW FODMAP

After sticking to this FoodFrame, you might be anxious to start eating a wider variety of foods, but you will get the best results only if you start to reintroduce in small amounts only one specific category at a time. *I can't impress this upon you enough*! If you dive into your old ways too soon, you will see symptoms return immediately. For example, you could start with a food you are really missing like avocados. Try one-quarter of an avocado or less and see how you do. If you don't have a reaction, try it again or maybe even increase the portion size to a half. If you continue to thrive, then stay at that portion every few days and then start to add some other food item. I highly encourage you to go slowly!

Once you begin to reintroduce foods, assess how you feel and how your body reacts. Keep a food diary, which will be extremely helpful for keeping track of what you eat and drink. If any of those foods are causing gastric upset, bloating, gas, constipation, or diarrhea, stop eating them for another few weeks and then slowly add them in again. Onions, garlic, and cauliflower are foods that I see affecting people for the long term. Sometimes people need to remove them completely or enjoy them on rare occasions. If at any time your symptoms return, feel free to restart the Low FODMAP FoodFrame from the beginning. If that happens, I recommend that you stay on it for a full four weeks for best results.

LOW FODMAP - RECIPES

Bluemania Shake

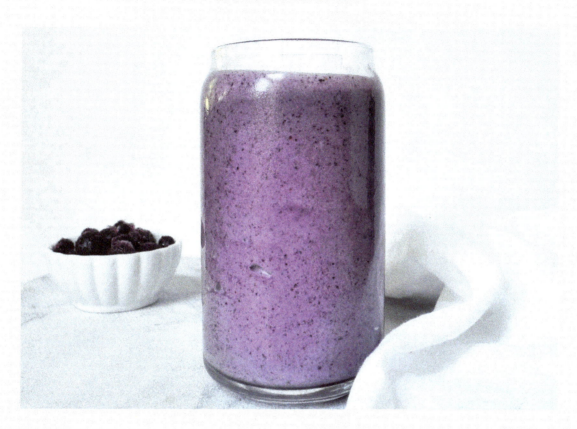

🍴 Ingredients:

1 cup coconut nut milk
10 macadamia nuts (raw or roasted, unsalted)
1 scoop RGN Collagen Protein, vanilla
1 cup frozen, organic blueberries

🍴 Instructions:

1. Place all ingredients in a blender and blend until smooth.
2. Garnish with unsweetened coconut shreds or shaved macadamia nuts.

Serves 1

Shakshuka

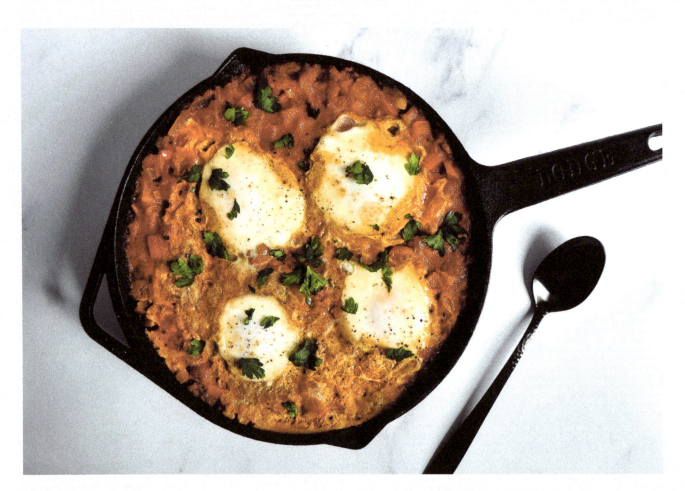

🍴 Ingredients:

2 tablespoons coconut oil
1 medium white or yellow onion, diced
1 large organic red bell pepper, diced
3 cloves garlic, minced
1 tablespoon tomato paste
1 teaspoon ground cumin
½ teaspoon smoked paprika

1 28-ounce can organic crushed tomatoes
2 tablespoons chopped fresh flat-leaf parsley, plus additional parsley leaves for garnish
Sea salt and ground black pepper to taste
5 to 6 large eggs

Instructions:

1. Heat coconut oil over medium heat in a large cast iron or regular skillet. Add the onion and bell pepper. Cook, stirring often, until the onions are tender and translucent, about 4 to 6 minutes.
2. Add garlic, tomato paste, cumin, and paprika. Cook, stirring constantly, about 1 to 2 minutes.
3. Pour in the crushed tomatoes with their juices, sea salt, pepper, and chopped parsley. Stir and let the mixture come to a simmer. Reduce the heat as necessary to maintain a gentle simmer and cook for 5 minutes to give the flavors time to meld.
4. Make slight divots in the sauce with the back of a large spoon, each equally distant from the other. Crack open the eggs and gently place one into a divot. Turn the heat to low and cover the pan.
5. Check the eggs after 4 minutes and cook until the whites of the eggs are fully cooked.
6. Sprinkle with a light dusting of sea salt and pepper.

Serves 2-4

Risa Groux, CN

Chicken Noodle Soup

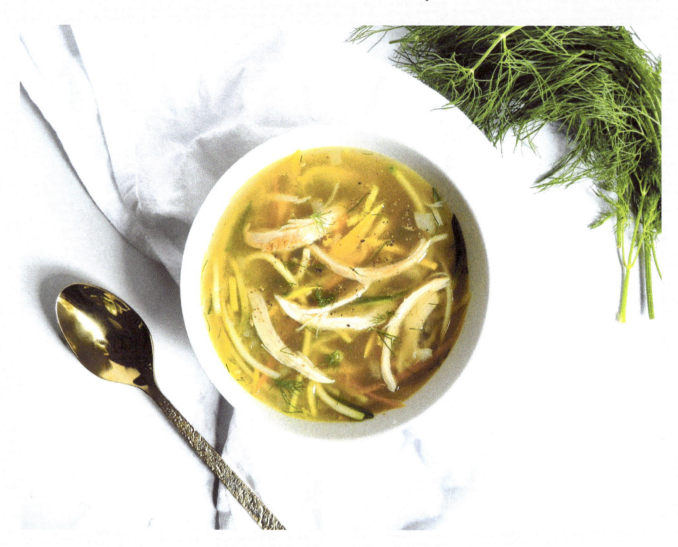

🍴 Ingredients:

4 cups chicken bone broth (I use Bonafide Provisions)
½ tablespoon coconut or grape seed oil
½ yellow onion, chopped
2 organic zucchinis, ends removed
3 long orange carrots, peeled with both tips removed
long parsnip, peeled with both tips removed
1-2 boneless chicken breast
¼ cup fresh dill, chopped

Sea salt and pepper to taste

Instructions:

1. Julienne with a mandolin or spiralize zucchini, carrots, and parsnips.
2. In a soup pot, heat oil over medium heat and add the chopped onion. Stir until onion is translucent. Add bone broth, chicken, zucchini, carrots, and parsnips.
3. Cook the chicken on medium-high heat until fully cooked, approximately 10-15 minutes. Remove chicken and pull into shreds or cut into bite-sized pieces.
4. Add shredded chicken to the soup pot along with dill, salt, and pepper. Let cook for another 5 minutes and serve.

Serves 4-6

Risa Groux, CN

Potato Chips

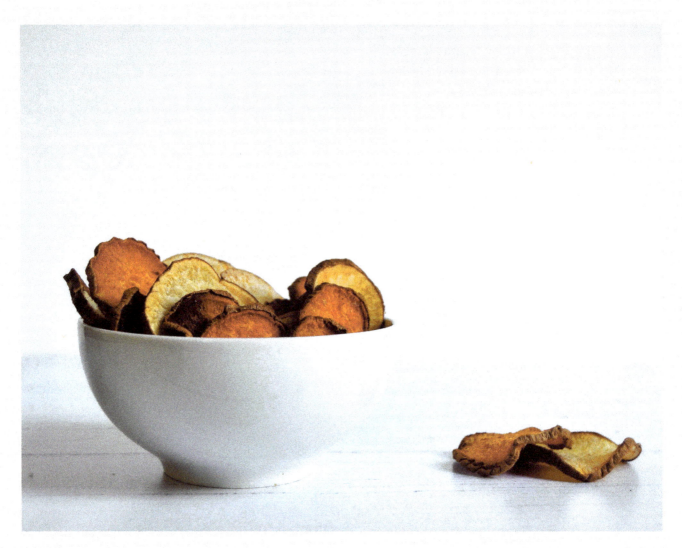

🍴 Ingredients:

2 potatoes (can be purple, sweet, or yam)
1-2 tablespoons olive oil
Sea salt to taste

🍴 Instructions:

Preheat oven to 350 degrees.

1. Scrub potatoes well but do not peel. Using a mandolin or knife, cut potatoes into thin rounds then place in large bowl. Add olive oil and lightly cover with sea salt.
2. Place on a cookie sheet and bake for approximately 30-45 minutes. Cooking time may vary depending on thickness of the potatoes and how crispy you like them. Turn chips half-way through baking time.

Optional: Use additional seasonings such as Cajun, paprika, or cinnamon.

Serves 4-6

Crispy Chicken Wings

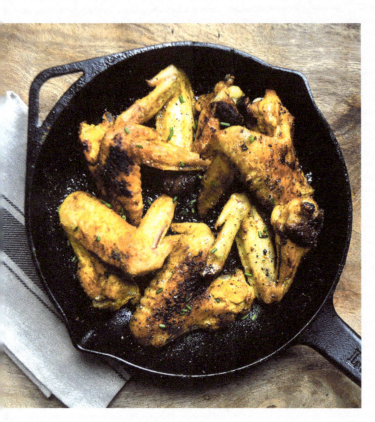

🍴 Ingredients:

12 raw chicken wings
1 tablespoon avocado oil
2 teaspoons ground ginger
2 teaspoons curry
2 teaspoons turmeric
Juice of ½ lemon
1 teaspoon black pepper
1 teaspoon sea salt

🍴 Instructions:

Preheat oven to 375 degrees.

1. Place chicken wings in a large bowl along with all the ingredients. Mix with your hands to ensure each wing is covered with the seasoning.
2. Place chicken wings in an ovenproof or cast-iron pan and cook on medium-high heat. If more oil is needed, add a little at a time. Turn wings until most of the skin is browned but not burnt.
3. Place skillet in the oven and cook for 35-45 minutes until crispy.

Makes 12 wings

Thai Salad with Sesame Ginger Dressing

Ingredients:

4 cups red leaf lettuce, washed and torn
1 cup of carrots, shredded
1 cup purple cabbage, shredded
1 cup Napa cabbage, shredded
1 cup cucumber, diced or julienned
1 cup cilantro, chopped
Sprinkle of black and white sesame seeds

Sesame Ginger Dressing:
½ cup sesame oil
2 tablespoons almond butter, unsweetened
½ cup coconut aminos
½-inch piece fresh ginger, peeled

Instructions:

For Sesame Ginger Dressing:
Place all ingredients in a food processor or blender and blend until smooth.

For Salad:
Place all salad ingredients in a bowl and toss with the dressing.

Optional: Add shredded chicken or shrimp.

Serves 4-6

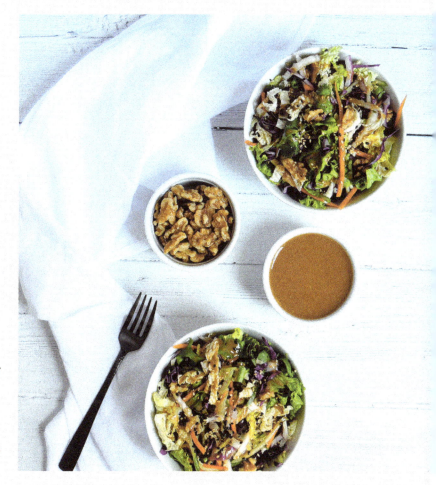

Zucchini Pasta with Pesto

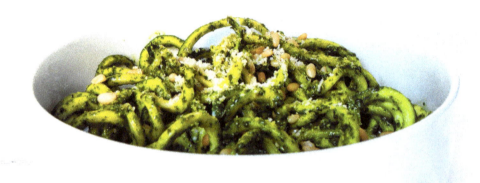

🍴 Ingredients:

4-6 zucchini, washed and spiralized
1 tablespoon coconut oil

Pesto:
½ cup olive oil or garlic infused olive oil
3 cups packed kale leaves, stems removed
1 cup packed fresh basil leaves
⅓ cup pine nuts or toasted walnuts
Sea salt and pepper to taste

Instructions:

1. Heat a large skillet on medium heat and melt the coconut oil. Place zucchini spirals in the pan and cook, stirring frequently to remove the moisture. Drain, place in a serving bowl, and set aside.
2. Place olive oil, kale and basil into a food processor and blend until smooth. Add pine nuts or walnuts, sea salt, and pepper to taste and blend again until smooth.
3. Combine the pesto with the zucchini and stir well to combine.

Optional: Top with grilled chicken, shrimp, or scallops and garnish with basil leaves or halved cherry tomatoes.

Serves 4

Whipped Parsnips

Ingredients:

3 large parsnips, peeled and trimmed
¾ cup coconut cream (hard cream from the top of coconut milk or use coconut cream)
Sea salt to taste
Garnish with parsley

Instructions:

1. Cut parsnips into chunks and steam for 10 minutes until soft.
2. Place steamed parsnips in a food processor or high-speed blender, add the coconut cream and a couple pinches of sea salt. Whip for about a minute until smooth. Add more salt if needed and garnish with parsley.

Serves 4

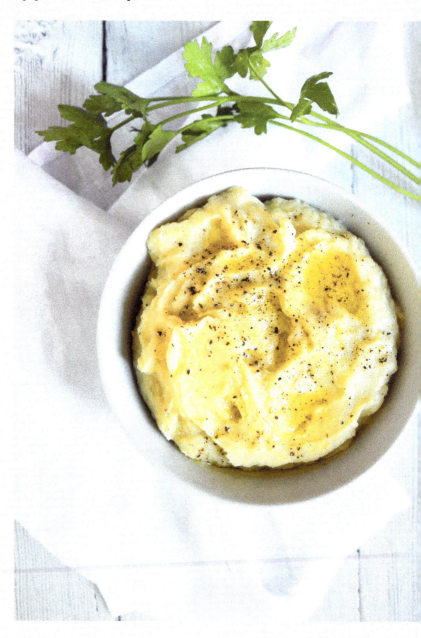

Coconut Cookies

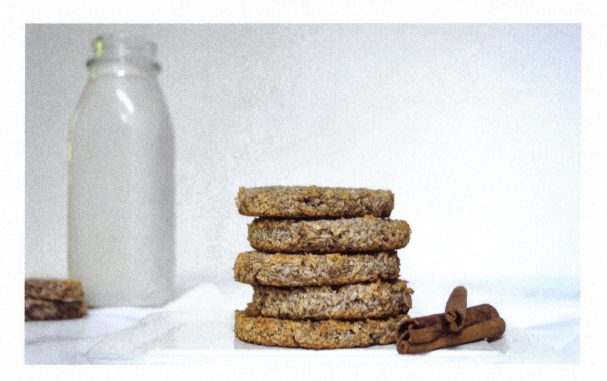

Ingredients:

2 ripe bananas
1½ cups unsweetened coconut shreds
1 teaspoon cinnamon

Instructions:

Preheat oven to 350 degrees. Line a cookie sheet with parchment paper and set aside.

1. Place bananas in a blender or mini chopper and blend until smooth. Transfer to a bowl and add coconut shreds and cinnamon. Mix until well combined.
2. Using a medium cookie scoop, make batter balls and place onto a cookie sheet. Evenly flatten with the back of a spatula to form into cookies.
3. Bake for 25 minutes or until golden brown.

Makes 9 cookies

Risa Groux, CN

Chocolate Collagen Pudding

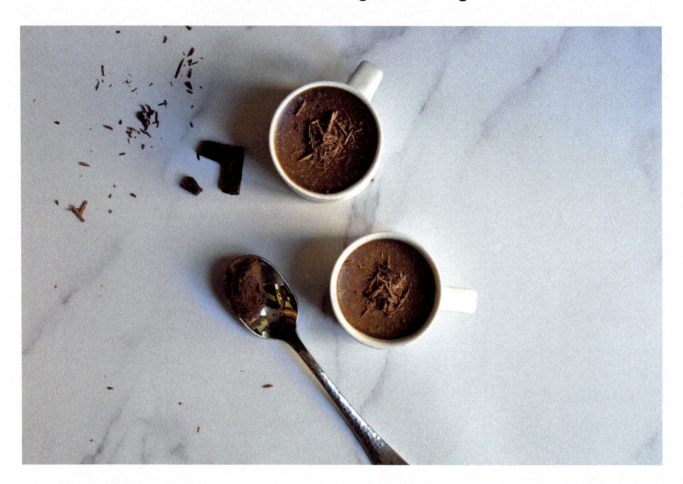

🍴 Ingredients:

2 (13.5oz) cans full fat coconut cream
4 scoops of RGN Collagen Protein, chocolate
2 tablespoons raw cacao powder (less if you prefer a less intense chocolate taste)
2 tablespoons almond butter
2 teaspoons monk fruit

Instructions:

1. Using an electric or hand-held mixer, mix all ingredients on medium speed for 6-8 minutes until smooth. Scrape down the sides if needed. Let it sit for a minute or two to let the mixture settle.
2. Pour into serving jars and place in the refrigerator for six or more hours.

Garnish and serve.

Makes 4-8 depending on the size of your servings.

EPILOGUE
LIFE BEYOND THE FOODFRAME

At this point, you have taken the FoodFrame quiz, perhaps had your blood drawn, and did a stool test. You should now have a fairly good idea of which FoodFrame best suits you based on your test results and health status. I encourage you to follow that course until you start thriving for at least a solid two months. To reap the highest rewards be attuned to how your body is reacting and stay in the box as much as you can.

If you would like to expand your eating lifestyle with choices outside your particular FoodFrame, try adding one food group at a time and see how your body responds. By now, you're much more conscious of how your body communicates with you, so watch for signs like an upset stomach, diarrhea, constipation, headaches, joint pain, bloating, and fatigue. If you experience any of those symptoms, then go back to the FoodFrame and give it another couple of months before attempting new foods again.

Regardless of the FoodFrame my clients follow, this is what I see in my practice:

- The vast majority do best leaving gluten and dairy out, however, some people can tolerate them in small doses. They are both inflammatory foods, so I recommend you enjoy them only on rare occasion, if you can tolerate them.
- The Paleo, Autoimmune Protocol, Low Lectin, and Vegetarian FoodFrames can all become a lifestyle rather than a short-term solution.
- Keto is great for three to four month stretches, but I think it is important to take a break from time to time.
- The Low FODMAP diet can be followed with some allowances, but if IBS, IBD, or SIBO symptoms return, then hop back on this diet. I know several people who mostly adhere to Low FODMAP as their SIBO is constantly recurring, nearly everyone who suffers from this condition feels best while following a Low FODMAP eating plan.
- The Risa Groux Nutrition Detox is a great reset that can be performed up to four times per year. Not only does it get the toxins out of the body, but it resets your palate for real whole food, and removes cravings for sugar, carbs, and processed foods. Weight loss is a great side effect!

Regardless of your FoodFrame, I encourage you to eat mostly for your health and occasionally for sport. Your body will let you know when you have gone too far. Now you have the tools to dial it back!

I sincerely hope you've found this book informative. Remember, what you've learned in these pages is not about a diet…it's about lifestyle.

I see people struggle with food every day and it kills me how much they don't know about the basic necessities of eating well for their health. None of us were taught properly. People everywhere struggle with their emotional relationship with food, diet confusion, and food choices--and with a million mixed messages out there, the confusion and frustration magnify.

No one diet fits all, which is why diet books don't work for everyone. This book gives you the power to explore which FoodFrame best fits you. I hope you can hear what your body tells you so you can make the best possible decisions to optimize your health with every meal!

ACKNOWLEDGMENTS

Every solid structure has a strong foundation. It takes a blueprint to build a solid structure from beginning to completion. I am so incredibly grateful to have a multitude of pillars in my life who have endlessly supported me with my passion for nutrition, natural health, quality food, and the birth of this book.

First and foremost, my children Sarah and Chase. Thank you both for being my full-time cheerleaders, watching every health documentary I ask you to, reading labels and the articles I send, and providing continuous encouragement and support. Sarah is responsible for making my life beautiful. She has helped create the soul of every gorgeous food photo, branding concepts, and social media accounts. I cannot possibly count the number of days we created, cooked, cleaned, and danced in the kitchen together, which brings me ultimate and absolute joy!

Chase has been incredibly patient trying all my new mealtime experiments. When he says, "Mom, this is good, but you don't need to make it again" I know my experiment did not make the cut. I love that you enjoy every vegetable, and you take your supplements…most of the time. I am over the top proud of you both! You care what goes into your bodies, minimize your toxic load, detox when needed, and value your health…I am so incredibly grateful for that! I wouldn't be where I am without you both!

Eric my almost-son, I am so proud of how you've embraced and value healthy eating, have your daily collagen shake, exercise regularly, and educated your fraternity that soda is poison. I just love how you and Sarah plan and cook healthy home cooked meals, even for Pesto, the cutest dog ever!

My parents have been a tremendous support throughout my childhood. Thank you both for cooking our meals with real ingredients, having family dinner most nights, and for making fast-food trips a very occasional treat and not an everyday thing. You gave me a love for real food and cooking from the beginning. I greatly appreciate your endless support, confidence, enthusiasm, and your belief in me! I cherish our time together!

I couldn't ask for better brothers! You and your families hold me up regularly in ways you don't even know. Thank you for letting me mess up your kitchens and feed your families.

I feel incredibly fortunate to have a million memories with both my grandmothers, especially in the kitchen! They weren't gourmet cooks, but a fresh healthy meal was always on tap with a heaping side dish of love, concern, support and loads of laughter. Roasted chicken, garbanzo beans in a salad, and matzo brei will remind me of you both for eternity.

Thank you to my powerhouse group of women whom I adore, respect, learn from, laugh and cry with, hike, walk, and bike with, confide in, and spend my free time with. I couldn't do this journey without you all. You have rooted for me from the very minute I wanted to become a nutritionist and have been excited to hold this book in your hands. Too many to mention names but you know who you are. From the bottom of my heart, I love you and thank you all.

Friends are the one of the essential pillars we need to ensure we thrive. I have attained quality friendships from every stage in life. Thank you for making me stretch, search, create, and cook with and for you. Bob, you have watched my passion for nutrition blossom for 25 years. Thank you for your support.

Thank you to Angelica Smith and Raechel Koob, who have been amazing to work with and bring organization and sanity to a very busy practice.

I am incredibly grateful to those in practice who have been abundantly generous to me in teaching me functional nutrition, encouraging me to keep learning through conferences and seminars, and everything about blood work! You enabled me to help so many and create a thriving practice of my own. Thank you, Paul Fisher, David Hallam, Dr. Michelle Hallam, Dr. Aaron Newman, and Dr. Frankie Scott-Cannova. Mendi Kessler, you gave me wings to soar.

Writing a book is a winding road. I have learned so much and am grateful to those who believe in me and helped pave the way: Dr. Josh Axe, Samantha Dunn, Dr. Stephen Gundry, JJ Virgin, Emily Loftiss, Elizabeth Much, Karen Murgolo, Karen Moline, L.E. Saba, and Suzanne Somers.

Thank you, Nancy Fries and Harry Karp, for all your grammar guidance and endless support!

To my needle Ron Miller, thank you for helping to stitch up the finishing touches!

And lastly, I want to thank all the clients I have worked with through the years in my practice who have trusted me to help them find their health and vitality. You mean the world to me and I truly enjoy working with you and watching you thrive!

APPENDIX I
Risa Groux Nutrition Supplements

I am very picky about what goes into my body, my loved one's bodies along with the bodies of everyone I work with. Too many supplements on the market are filled with artificial ingredients, dyes, additives, preservatives, and even processed oils that can cause inflammation, more harm than the benefit it was intended to create.

I am committed to producing the highest quality, purity, potency, using efficacious nutrients. I look to scientific research before creating any and all RGN products to ensure an effective and safe product.

All RGN products are evaluated and monitored for potential contaminants such as heavy metals and pesticides while ensuring compliance with FDA Good Manufacturing Practices (GMPs). In addition, all RGN products are gluten, dairy, soy, and sugar free as well as Non-GMO. The RGN product line consists of:

Foods/Edible Nutrients	**Description**	**Benefits**
Collagen Protein Powder (chocolate & vanilla)	Collagen protein powder; great for making shakes or baking	Supports gut healing, joints, connective tissue, immunity, beneficial for hair, skin, and nails, and cellulite
Collagen Paleo Chocolate Bars	Protein bars that are a great meal replacement or snack	Supports gut health, joints, connective tissue, immune system, and hair, skin & nails
Immune Ultra Lozenges	Zinc and elderberry lozenges	Promotes immunity
Gut Reboot Powder	L-glutamine, zinc carnicine, Slippery elm, marshmallow root	Supports gut healing and the integrity of intestinal lining

Detoxes:

14-Day Whole Food Detox	Collagen protein powder and detox/antioxidant capsules for 14 days, along with a food plan booklet	Promotes detoxification, which will benefit in weight loss, mental clarity, increased energy, decreased joint pain, headaches/migraines, increased gut health and decreased inflammation.
14-Day Plant-Based Detox	Plant-based protein powder and detox/antioxidant capsules for 14 days, along with a food plan booklet	Promotes detoxification, which will benefit in weight loss, mental clarity, increased energy, decreased joint pain, headaches/migraines, increased gut health and decreased inflammation

Supplements:

D3 Ultra with K	Vitamin D3 with Vitamin K for maximum absorption	Maintenance and support of the immune system, brain, bone, thyroid, gut, and nervous system
B Ultra	Methylated B complex, Including B12, folate, and biotin	Increases energy; helps combat stress, supports intestinal lining
Enzyme Max	Digestive enzymes for proteins, fats, and carbohydrates	Improves digestion and reduces bloating/gastric upset. Includes all pancreatic enzymes, HCL, and ox bile
Magnesium	300 mg buffered chelated magnesium per 2 capsules	Supports proper function of nerves, muscles, cells, and tissue; supports bone health and sleep
Omega Max	600 mg EPA and 400 mg DHA in each two soft gel serving	Promotes brain, heart, and eye health; decreases inflammation

Turmeric Max	330 mg of high dose curcumin	Anti-inflammatory, pain reliever, anti-oxidant power to quench free radical damage
PostBio Max	Short-chain fatty acids	Gut healing; Feeds the colon its essential food source, provides diversity of the microbiome
RGN Weight Loss Support	60 packets for a 30-day supply. Each packet contains 5 capsules with all natural ingredients such as L-Carnitine, Garcinia Extract, Chromium and other nutrients	Curbs cravings, Promotes efficient metabolism, Supports focused eating
Adrenal Reboot	Standardized adaptogenic herbs and nutrients	Helps support healthy cortisol levels, hypothalamic and pituitary function, and catecholamine production
Ultra Calm	GABA, L-theanine, 5-HTP, and chamomile	Helps support healthy mood, cravings, and feelings of calm, satiety, and satisfaction
Berberine Balance	Highly BioAvaliable Berberine	Supports healthy blood sugar levels and enhancing insulin sensitivity

APPENDIX II
Most Commonly Ordered Tests

Most Commonly Ordered Tests

Lab	Tests
Diagnostic Solutions (877) 485-5336	GI Map
Lab Corp (800) 845-6167	Comprehensive Bio Screen MTHFR Epstein Barr Virus (EBV) Cytomegalovirus (CMV) Hormone panels
Direct Labs (800) 908-0000	MTHFR Hormone panels
DiagnosTechs (425) 251-0596	Adrenal Stress Index (ASI). Expanded Female Hormone Panel (Saliva)
Cyrex Laboratories (602) 759-1245	Array 2 (Intestinal Antigenic Permeability Screen) Array 3X (Wheat/Gluten Proteome Reactivity and Autoimmune) Array 4 (Gluten Associated Cross Reactive Foods and Foods Sensitivity) Array 5 (Multiple Autoimmune Reactivity Screen) Array 10 (Multiple Food Immune Reactivity Screen)

CPSIA information can be obtained
at www.ICGtesting.com
Printed in the USA
LVHW071652240122
709251LV00019B/694